D1599475

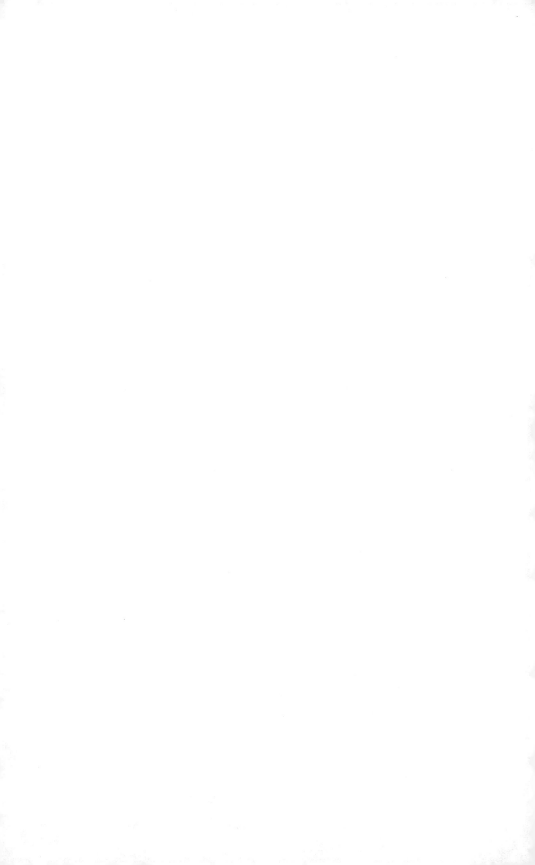

Intermittent Fasting for Women Over 50

The One-Stop Guide to Lose Weight, Slow Down Aging, and Support Your Hormones While Still Enjoying Delicious Meals and Social Gatherings

Contents

Introduction

Intermittent fasting (IF) was named the "trendiest" weight loss term searched on Google in 2019 and was featured in the New England Journal of Medicine. These two things happened for a reason. This diet method had quickly become one of the most popular among dieters. Anyone who is a part of the weight loss and fitness world likely knows what it entails.

Intermittent fasting involves alternate fasting and eating cycles. You have periods when you eat and periods when you fast. There have been many proven benefits, such as weight loss, health improvement, and disease protection. Another possible advantage is that it could help you live longer.

Naturally, there are tons of resources available online to teach people how to practice intermittent fasting. Still, not all these resources include factual information that can improve your health and life quality. This is precisely why Intermittent Fasting for Women over 50 exists. This book has been written explicitly to target women in their 50s or their menopausal stage of life.

It is common knowledge that weight loss generally becomes more challenging once you reach a specific age. Why does that happen? How can intermittent fasting help solve the problem? Can intermittent fasting help achieve healthy weight loss? Can you slow aging with this dieting method? These are a few questions you will find concise answers to in this book.

It contains up-to-date information compared to many other books on the market. It is written in simple and straightforward language to ease understanding. It breaks down the most complex terms to make for fluid assimilation. What sets it apart from other books is that it contains practical, hands-on instructions and techniques you can instantly incorporate into your daily routine.

With this book, you can start your intermittent fasting journey with confidence, knowing you have a practical and reliable guide to achieve your weight loss goals.

Chapter One: Why Dieting Isn't Easy Over 50

"Why am I gaining weight without making changes to my dieting or exercise routine?"

The above is a question that women in their 50s often have to ask their doctors. Gaining weight without eating more or exercising less can be heartbreaking for anybody, but women are more likely to be affected.

As a woman in your 50s, you want to look as good and fit as you always have. You don't expect your age to affect anything. But to your dismay, it is affecting everything. You are gaining more weight than you want. And even though you are exercising and doing all you can to lose the extra fat, it seems like your efforts are futile.

The scenario painted above is something that anyone, men or women, over 50 can relate to, regardless of background differences. Losing weight becomes harder for most people once they reach a certain age. Aging comes with many things that cumulate to significantly inhibit weight loss, enough for you to observe that changes are happening within your body.

Suppose you have been dieting and exercising without seeing expected results. There, it means that your body is experiencing age-related changes, which may be sabotaging your efforts. As you age, you lose lean muscle mass. This results in a slower metabolism. Understandably, your physical activity also decreases, leading to reduced calorie burning.

Even if you are a fit person, you are bound to experience these alterations between the ages of 40 and 50. That is when you notice the weight gain creeping in on you gradually. You might have lost weight by cutting out a snack from your diet. But now, doing that changes nothing.

The older you get, the less your body responds to weight loss efforts. A review by the Agency for Healthcare Research and Quality explains that people gain 1 to 2 pounds every year as they age. At first, you may think this isn't much, but the result is significant weight gain over time. In a few cases, it may even lead to obesity.

Not everyone adds pounds to the point where they become overweight. Genetic makeup, physical activity level, and dietary choices are a few things that influence body weight. Still, everyone struggles with weight loss or maintenance as they get older. The difference lies in how much weight you gain.

Before we go deep into the different reasons why older people, especially women, find it harder to lose or maintain weight, I want to address a common misconception. The misconception is that men lose weight faster than women and are not affected by the age-related issues in their fifties, which is misleading.

Men, like women, also experience difficulty with weight loss and maintenance the older they get. People commonly believe that men have an advantage over women in matters of weight loss. Well, this is somewhat true, but there is a catch.

Men burn more calories than body fat because they have more lean muscle tissue than women. So, even when a man is resting and not indulging in any physical activity, he can lose weight. And when a man and a woman cut the same amounts of calories from their diets, the man still loses more weight.

It is why many people believe that men have an advantage over women. But this doesn't work out in the long run. Over the long term, both genders get an equal playing field. The main difference is that men do not undergo the same hormonal changes as women do.

When you reach the menopausal age range, estrogen production reduces to a considerable extent. The sudden decrease in estrogen levels results in transferring fat to your midsection, which consequentially increases the risk of stroke, type 2 diabetes, heart disease, and other conditions.

As a woman in your 50s, there are several reasons you might find it difficult to lose or maintain your weight.

The first reason is due to losing muscle due to age. After the age of 30, your lean muscle mass naturally declines by up to 8 percent per decade. According to a publication in the Current Opinion in Clinical Nutrition and Metabolic Care, researchers call this process sarcopenia.

Age-related conditions such as arthritis often result in reduced physical activity, which, in turn, leads to muscle loss. Another possible cause of muscle loss is prolonged injury. Individually, none of these causes significant muscle loss. But together, they make a substantial impact.

Now, you might be wondering what this has to do with you exercising, dieting, and losing weight. Well, lean muscle puts more calories to work than fat. Unless you regularly engage in strength-based exercises to build and maintain your muscles, your body will require fewer calories daily. That makes you more likely to gain weight if you keep consuming the same number of calories you did when you were younger.

Most women don't realize this, so they don't bother adjusting the calories in their diets. They continue eating the usual amount, but they find it difficult to burn calories with muscle loss. Combine this with reduced physical activities, and you have several pounds gained over time.

Another reason you may find weight loss in your 50s difficult is because of hormonal changes. As a woman, you experience specific changes that are normal and natural. Even men undergo these changes as well but in different ways. It is a part of the aging process. It explains why the Center for Disease Control's scientific data shows that middle age is the prime time for weight gain.

Menopause triggers a significant drop in your estrogen levels when you are between 45 and 55. It allows you to gain extra pounds around your belly area. Usually, the shift in fat location makes your weight gain more noticeable. It also increases your risk of developing heart disease, high cholesterol, high blood pressure, and type 2 diabetes.

And there is something called *perimenopause,* the period leading up to menopausal age. During this period, you might experience mood fluctuations, making it challenging to conform to healthy eating and exercise. Due to this, you may gain about five pounds during the transition from perimenopause to menopause.

In contrast, men start experiencing a dip in testosterone levels around 40 years old. This happens at a rate of about 1 to 2 percent every year. Testosterone in men is responsible for muscle strength, muscle mass, and fat distribution regulation. A decline in its production naturally affects all of these functions, reducing the body's effectiveness at burning calories.

Also, the growth hormone (GH) production reduces in both men and women, which further affects the body. Among other things, the growth hormone's function is to build muscle mass. It is also responsible for maintenance. So, the more it declines, the harder your body finds it to develop and maintain muscle mass. Inadvertently, this impacts the number of calories your body can effectively burn.

You accumulate more fat, build less lean muscle mass, burn fewer calories, and this continues over time. It keeps adding up, resulting in a snowball effect for your weight loss and maintenance journey.

Because of the decline in muscle mass building and maintenance, metabolism becomes slower than ever. That is another likely reason losing weight at your older age seems almost impossible. As you may already know, metabolism is a complex process that converts calories into energy inside your body.

When you have less muscle and more fat, your body burns calories slower. Remember that exercise is one way your body boosts metabolism. So, as you become less physically active at this age, your metabolism automatically becomes slower than before.

Your age isn't the only thing that impacts your metabolic rate. Sex and body size play vital roles, too. Some health conditions may also affect your metabolism. An example of such a condition is hypothyroidism.

By the time you are in your late forties and early fifties, you are likely at the peak of your career. While this is great, it poses significant weight loss challenges to you. To begin with, you may be moving less than you did when you were younger.

Maybe you spend an hour commuting to and from work and then spend up to eight hours seated at a desk every day, except weekends. You may also have a lot on your plate to where you can't spare enough time for a brisk walk or workout during the week.

To take it further, you may find you are too busy to take a lunch break most days, increasing your chances of getting calorie-condensed food from the vending machine. Ultimately, you may become subject to increased work-related stress. A study by Jen-Chieh Chuang and Jeffrey M. Zigman on Ghrelin's Roles in Stress, Mood, and Anxiety Regulation published in the International Journal of Peptides in 2010 suggests that work-related stress increases ghrelin production levels and that can make you hungrier.

Women experience significant life changes between the ages of 40 and 50, resulting in weight gain. Sometimes, you gain weight because of what is going on in your life, not the things happening within your body.

One of the most significant changes you may experience in your thirties is the start of a family. When you have a new family, the hours you spend at the gym may suddenly seem like they are more productive if you invest them in your toddler.

And you even have to engage in several parenting activities such as going on playdates, getting the homework done, and many other activities that require your undivided attention. It may seem like you don't have time for yourself anymore. Due to this, your diet and exercise routine might slip, causing you to add a few pounds.

As you have likely noticed, this chapter is merely to give you a deep insight into why weight loss isn't easy for women like you. The next chapter will reveal the basics of intermittent fasting. More important, you will discover how it can serve as your solution to these age-related issues that hinder your fitness journey.

So, let's get right to it!

Chapter Two: How Does Intermittent Fasting Work?

First, intermittent fasting is not a fad. You may find this unbelievable considering how trendy it has been for the past few years, but it is more than just another trend. Researchers and scientists have been studying this dieting strategy in laboratories around the world. Nobody invests valuable resources in what they believe to be a fad. Therefore, the first perception you should have of IF is that it is real, and it works.

Intermittent fasting is a dieting strategy that involves restricting "when" you eat to cut down your calorie intake. Unlike other dieting strategies, intermittent fasting has little to do with what you eat. Contrary to assumptions, it doesn't mean you have to starve yourself to lose weight. It doesn't give you a pass to consume as many unhealthy foods as you want, either.

The basis is that you eat within specific windows of time instead of eating different meals and snacks throughout the day. You may also call it periodic eating.

Unlike actual fasting, where you consume no meals or snacks within a specified period, intermittent fasting allows you to eat to an extent. It focuses on when to eat rather than what to eat.

Not consuming any calories for a specified number of hours per day or week can help your body burn fat more quickly and efficiently. Scientific studies suggest there are certain health benefits you can gain from fasting. An excellent example is a study titled "*Effect of Intermittent Fasting on Health, Aging, and* Disease" by De Cabo R and Mattson MP, published in the England Journal of Medicine in 2019. Calorie and mealtime restrictions can help with weight loss. But that is not all – it also reduces the risk of different diseases.

Some fasting schedules require you to fast up to 18 hours each day. It all depends on the fasting schedule you choose. In your fasting window, you do not eat anything that could increase your calorie intake. Then you can consume calories during the eating window.

The best thing about the fasting window is that it is not as difficult as it sounds. It often falls at bedtime, so most people sleep for about eight of the fasting hours. Additionally, you can consume non-calorie drinks such as coffee, tea, and water, making the whole process relatively easy for the average person.

There are several ways you can try intermittent fasting. Still, the basis of all the methods is that you choose regular periods to eat and fast. For example, you might eat during a six-hour window every day and then fast for the rest of the day. You might also choose a 24-hour fasting window after which you eat for the following 24-hour period. The point is that there are varying fasting schedules. The subsequent chapter delves deeper into the plans and shows you how you can choose one that works for you.

Most Americans eat throughout their waking hours, which is a stark contrast to the intermittent fasting eating pattern. If you eat three meals a day, with snacks, and little to no exercise, it means you are running on calories every time you eat. Simply put, you are not burning fat from your fat stores. Periodic fasting changes this unhelpful pattern by prolonging the time when your body burns through consumed calories from your last meal and starts burning your fat stores.

As you will have gathered, this dieting strategy is more about when you eat than what you eat. During your fasting window, you can consume zero-calorie beverages. And during the eating window, you only need to eat normally. You don't have to change what you eat. You still have the liberty to consume your favorite regular foods.

You shouldn't binge-eat to compensate for the fasting periods. You are unlikely to achieve your weight loss goals or become healthier if you pack your eating window with all kinds of high-calorie junk.

Many people like intermittent fasting because it does not limit them from enjoying any food they want. It teaches you to be mindful of when you eat to promote better health and fitness, but it gives no restrictions on the kinds of food to eat. Just remember that you still have to eat healthy when fasting.

Intermittent fasting is ideal for you or any woman in her fifties for several reasons. The main reason is that the limited eating window naturally limits the calories you consume every day. The previous chapter stated that weight loss becomes a challenge in the fifties because women continue to consume the same number of calories they did at a younger age. Still, the body finds them harder to burn.

When you start fasting, your calorie intake automatically reduces, which means that your body has fewer calories to burn. The fewer calories consumed, the easier the body can burn fat.

The benefits of intermittent fasting are not limited to calorie restriction, particularly for older women. Many experts disagree with those who believe that IF works only because it limits food intake. These experts believe that the results people get from periodic fasting are much better than general meal schedules that involve consuming the same number of calories and other nutrients.

Some experts also suggest that daily food abstinence for several hours does not just restrict calorie consumption – it does more than that. Time-restricted fasting causes specific metabolic changes in the body. These changes account for some of its synergistic benefits.

The three changes are:

- **Insulin:** During your fasting window, insulin levels drop to encourage fat burning.

- **HGH**: As insulin levels drop, your HGH levels rise to improve muscle growth and fat burning.

- **Noradrenaline:** In response to fasting, your nervous system releases noradrenaline to your cells to inform them they need to burn fat for fuel

These changes cumulate to cause "metabolic switching," which scientists believe to be responsible for intermittent fasting benefits. Metabolic switching is simply when your body depletes its glycogen supply within 10 to 12 hours of fasting, after which it burns ketones. That is a sort of fuel that your liver makes from stored fat.

The switch from glycogen to ketones affects other chemicals in your body and your immune signals and growth factors. But ketones are not the only thing that happens. The periodic fasting and eating windows also activate genes and signaling pathways, making your neurons stronger.

Before we go deep into how intermittent fasting may be beneficial specifically to women in their 50s, here are a few evidence-based advantages according to science.

1. Changes in Cells, Genes, and Hormones Functions

One of the scientifically proven advantages of intermittent fasting is that it changes how your cells, genes, and hormones function. Several things happen in the body during the fasting window. For one, your body triggers some vital cellular repair processes. It also changes your hormone levels to make your body fat storage more accessible.

Insulin levels drop significantly, initiating the fat-burning process. The growth hormone production also increases as much as five-fold. As noted previously, increment in the production of this hormone facilitates muscle gain and fat burning. There are tons of other health benefits.

When you put off eating for a while, your body also repairs your cells. For example, it naturally removes waste materials from your cellular organs. Changes further occur through gene expression. Some changes contribute to protection against disease and longevity.

Most benefits associated with intermittent fasting result from hormones, cell functions, and gene expression changes.

2. Burns Belly Fat

The midsection is possibly the one place where women find it hardest to burn fat. Even in your twenties and thirties, losing belly fat is hard enough. But when you become older, it becomes even more challenging. Intermittent fasting can make it easy for you because it makes you eat fewer meals and snacks. Most people that try intermittent fasting end up taking in fewer calories unless they eat much more than they should during their eating windows.

The changes in hormone function resulting from fasting facilitate the foundation for fat burning and weight loss. Reduced insulin levels, increased growth hormone production, and higher noradrenaline levels all enhance the body's ability to break fat down, facilitating an opening to convert to energy.

Due to this, periodic fasting accelerates your metabolic rate by up to 14 percent, helping you burn even more calories than you usually do. Intermittent fasting helps on both sides of the calorie equation. It increases your metabolic rate and therefore boosts calorie-burning. It also reduces food intake and, thus, decreases calorie consumption.

Based on a review of the scientific literature, you can lose up to 8 percent of your weight over 24 weeks by fasting intermittently. This is a substantial amount of weight loss. Since metabolism generally slows as a person ages, intermittent fasting is key to increasing your metabolic rate and burning as many calories as you want.

The review further shows that intermittent fasting ensures less muscle loss than other calorie restriction methods. This means it can help reduce the loss of muscle that occurs to women in their fifties.

Considering all of these, you can tell that intermittent fasting is a powerful weight loss technique.

3. Reduces Type 2 Diabetes Risk

Intermittent fasting has been proven to reduce insulin resistance, which lowers your risk of developing type 2 diabetes. In the last few decades, type 2 diabetes has become common among Americans. Higher blood sugar levels are the highlight in the context of insulin resistance.

Anything that can help you reduce insulin resistance will inadvertently lower blood sugar levels and lower type 2 diabetes risk. Not surprisingly, the study mentioned earlier also shows that intermittent fasting is incredibly beneficial to improving insulin resistance and lowering blood sugar levels. The evidence shows that the benefits are impressive.

Through fasting, up to six percent of blood sugar levels are reduced, while insulin is reduced by up to thirty-one percent. So, if you at risk of developing the condition, intermittent fasting can do much more than help you burn fat.

4. De-Escalates Stress and Inflammation

Oxidative stress contributes to aging and different chronic diseases. It is triggered when free radicals, which are unstable molecules in the body, react with other vital molecules, resulting in damage. Several studies on the benefits of intermittent fasting have shown that it can boost the body's ability to resist oxidative stress.

Besides, the studies also show that intermittent fasting helps in the fight against inflammation. Medically inclined people know that inflammation is the number one driver of all kinds of common diseases.

Oxidative stress and inflammation tend to affect older people more than younger ones. Fasting periodically is a proven way to protect yourself against the aging process and improve your body's immunity against diseases.

5. Improves Heart Health

All over the world, heart disease is recognized as the most significant cause of death. There are various factors associated with the risk of heart disease. Evidence suggests that intermittent fasting improves these health markers. Some of them include blood pressure, blood sugar levels, inflammatory markers, LDL cholesterol, and blood triglycerides.

Most of the evidence comes from research done on animals. Further studies need to be done on the effect of heart disease in humans. But even the potential is exciting.

6. Autophagy

When you fast, your body triggers something known as autophagy. It is the process through which your body gets rid of waste from the cells. It involves your cells breaking down and metabolizing any dysfunctional and broken proteins built up in the cells over time. When this happens, your protection against diseases such as cancer and Alzheimer's disease increases.

Other benefits of intermittent fasting include:

- Improvement of physical performance
- Enhanced thinking and memory abilities
- Prevention of diabetes and obesity
- Decreased tissue damage

You are probably curious about how intermittent fasting can enhance your body's ability to burn calories and fat.

As explained earlier, decreased metabolism is one of the affective factors for challenging weight loss in older women. Most women are aware of this. When metabolism slows down, you find it harder to burn calories, which makes you add more pounds. With intermittent fasting, you can cut down the calories you consume to shed excess weight or even keep it off.

On average, a woman needs to cut at least 100 calories from her daily diet. Once you are in your 50s, the first step should be to cut your calorie intake from 1,800 daily to 1,600 per day. If you keep consuming 1,800 calories, you may add up to 10 pounds every year.

Intermittent fasting can help you cut down your calorie intake so you don't consume more than your body can effectively burn. You might like using IF to reduce calorie intake because you don't have to deprive yourself of certain foods. You can still eat what you want, but if specific foods add more calories than necessary to your diet, giving them up will help your journey.

Another problem mentioned in chapter one was reduced physical activity. How can intermittent fasting help with that? Well, it would be illogical to say that fasting can completely replace exercise and physical activity, but it can contribute.

Like fasting, exercise also triggers autophagy because it is key to cell regeneration. It does more than that, though. Autophagy helps to cleanse the body to optimize it, making fat-burning easier than ever. This process ensues in many benefits for you. Among these are building insulin resistance and slowing the aging process. Without autophagy, you may become prone to weight gain, higher cholesterol, and impaired brain function.

Autophagy is triggered by positive stress, which you get from exercising and engaging in tasking physical activities. Skipping meals is another way you can cause positive stress and, ultimately, initiate your body's autophagy process.

So, even if your activities are reduced due to age, fasting periodically can serve the same purpose. But fasting cannot serve as a total replacement for exercise. You still need to work out. Exercising has tons of other benefits that you cannot get from fasting. The best thing is to combine both to get the best result.

Activities such as walking, jogging, and swimming are easy on the lower back and knees, making them ideal for older people. Both are also effective for jump-starting metabolism and burning calories. We'll discuss this more in a subsequent chapter.

Sarcopenia, as you have learned, is the loss of muscle mass. It is a natural side-effect of the aging process. Intermittent fasting can be useful to combat muscle loss in less active adults. Age-induced muscle loss may be inevitable, but it's manageable if approached in the right way.

Without exercise or intense physical activity, weight loss typically occurs due to losing lean mass and fat mass. Your muscles are a part of your lean mass. Everything in your body, except fat, is part of your lean mass.

When you try any diet targeted at weight loss, you are likely to lose your lean mass. That shows that dieting methods, including intermittent fasting, may cause loss of muscle mass. Some studies have shown that intermittent fasting causes one to lose up to 2 pounds of lean mass, but other studies showed contrasting results.

This has led many researchers to suggest that intermittent fasting likely affects lean mass maintenance during weight loss more than other non-fasting diets. Although extensive research has not been done on this, it does show that the effect can vary from person to person.

Overall, the consensus is that periodic fasting does not cause more muscle loss than other types of diets. If you combine mild exercises with intermittent fasting, you can successfully reduce the rate of muscle mass loss. Intermittent fasting cannot be used to gain muscle. But if done the right way, it's used to reduce the loss.

Strength-training exercises are the best way to reduce the consistent loss of muscle in your older age. Doing pushups a few times a week while fasting intermittently can make all the difference you want in your weight loss journey. Note that strength-training may also prevent bone loss, another primary concern for any woman in her fifties.

There are several ways intermittent fasting counters the issues that could make weight loss more difficult for you in your older years. These are just a few of the important ones you should know.

Ultimately, the most exciting benefit of this dieting strategy is that it could potentially extend your lifespan. In other words, it can help boost longevity for its practitioners. Studies done on rats suggest that IF improves longevity as continuous calorie restriction does.

Several results of the studies conducted were dramatic. One study showed that rats that fasted periodically lived up to 83% longer than those that didn't fast.

While this study has not been replicated with humans, it confirms that IF may have anti-aging benefits for older people.

Considering the many known benefits due to metabolic switching and other health markers, intermittent fasting will help you do much more than lose weight. It can affect the quality of your health and life. Automatically reducing your calorie intake can help you lose weight and live a healthier and longer life.

Healthy eating is simple, but it is also challenging to maintain. One of the many obstacles is that you have to put in maximum effort to plan and cook healthy meals. Intermittent fasting is your key to easy dieting because it does not require you to prepare, cook, and clean up as many meals as you did before.

For this very reason, its popularity among fitness and weight enthusiast continues to grow. By incorporating it into your everyday dieting routine, you can lose weight and improve your health while living a simple life simultaneously.

Throughout the remaining chapters, you will discover more about why intermittent fasting has become a popular trend among life-hackers. Read on.

Chapter Three: Types of Intermittent Fasting Plans

Depending on your lifestyle and weight loss goals, there are several patterns of fasting to follow. Individually, every single method is effective, but if you don't figure out which one is more suitable for you, the results may not be as impressive as you want.

The difference in intermittent fasting methods lies in the calorie allowances and the number of fasting hours. The experience you get from this dieting method is affected wholly by you. There are seven ways you can fast intermittently. To help decide which is more appropriate, this chapter unravels the science and research behind each type of fasting and, more importantly, how you can maintain the diet you choose.

The 12:12 Plan

This is an intermittent fasting pattern where you fast for 12 hours and eat for the other 12 hours every day. For beginners, the 12:12 plan is one of the easiest methods to start with. It requires you to restrict your daily food and calorie intake to within a 12-hour eating window rather than eating throughout the day.

Once your 12-hour eating window is gone, you are not advised to consume anything that might give your body calories. Your options are limited to zero-calorie drinks like water and black coffee. Fasting for just 12 hours every day is all you need to reap the fantastic benefits of this dieting strategy.

The rules for this method are simple. You need to choose a 12-hour fasting window you can adhere to every day for as long as you plan to fast. This plan has a relatively small fasting window, which typically falls into sleep time. You can consume a specific number of calories each day without having to worry about burning fat.

The easiest way you can follow this plan is to make sure that your sleep time is included in your fasting window. For example, you may fast between 8 p.m. and 8 a.m. To adhere to this timeframe, you would have to finish dinner every day before 8 p.m. and wait until 7 a.m. before you can eat another meal. Naturally, you would be asleep for much of the time between your eating and fasting window.

Fasting for 12 hours is the lowest you can do, as that is when your body can trigger metabolic switching to burn fat for fuel. After you become familiar with fasting and the feeling within your body, you can swiftly change from this beginner plan to a more advanced one.

The longer the hours in your fasting window, the more fat your body can burn after metabolic switching occurs.

The 16:8 Plan

This particular method is one of the most popular plans among intermittent fasting enthusiasts. Some even believe it to be the most effective. The 16:8 plan involves fasting every day for 16 hours while limiting your eating window to 8 hours. Even though the eating window may look relatively small, you can still fit in two to three meals within your eating window. Martin Berkhan, a fitness expert, popularized the 16:8 plan, and several people call it the Lean Gains Protocol.

16:8 intermittent fasting pattern works by supporting your body's circadian rhythm, which you may also call its internal clock. Following this plan means you abstain from food at night and part of the morning and afternoon. The eating period tends to start at midday.

As with other types of IF patterns, you have no restrictions on the types of foods you can eat during the eating window. There are also no restrictions on the amount of food to eat. Still, you are generally advised to consume the same amount you usually do during mealtime. The flexibility of this method explains why most people find it relatively easy to follow.

The simplest way to follow this plan is to choose a fasting window that includes the time you sleep. Some IF experts suggest that fasters should finish all food intake in the early evening, possibly around 6 to 7 p.m. Metabolism typically slows down after early evening, although this approach may not be feasible for everyone.

Your daily routine may make it impossible for you to consume your evening meal until later. You need to avoid food for at least 2 hours before your bedtime. Below are a few 8-hour eating windows from which you can choose:

- 9 a.m. to 5 p.m.
- Noon to 8 p.m.
- 10 a.m. to 6 p.m.

Within these timeframes, you can eat and snack conveniently. Regular healthy eating is vital to prevent peaks and dips in blood sugar levels and to reduce the possibility of excessive hunger. If you have to, don't be afraid to experiment with different timeframes to figure out the best eating and fasting window for your lifestyle.

To maximize the potential benefits of the 16:8 diet, you must stick to nutritious foods and beverages during your eating period. Don't see fasting as an opportunity to consume as many junk foods as possible. Fill up your diet with nutrient-rich foods to round it out and gain the benefits of periodic fasting.

Although it has many health benefits, restricting yourself to an 8-hour window has drawbacks, and this means it may not be right for you. The restriction on food intake can push you to eat more than usual during your eating window. Subconsciously try to make up for hours expended on fasting without realizing it.

Rather than help you shed extra pounds, this may cause more weight gain, digestive problems and even cause you to develop unhealthy eating habits. Suppose you don't choose a timeframe that fits right into your daily routine. There, this fasting plan may also cause adverse short-term effects such as fatigue, hunger, and weakness. These typically subside once your body gets more familiar with the new routine.

The 5:2 Plan

Also called the fast diet, this plan is the most popular intermittent fasting method according to current trends. Michael Mosley, a British journalist, is responsible for popularizing the 5:2 technique. The name derives from the fasting pattern involving eating for five days of the week and fasting for the remaining two days.

You need not fast for two entire days. The idea is to restrict calorie intake to just 1200 calories on both days. This means you must not consume over 600 calories per day. Even though this method may seem like a lot, most people agree that it is easier to stick to than any other calorie-restricted diet.

Typically, you can eat for your 5-day eating window without restricting yourself to any specific amounts of calories. Then, within the two-day fasting window, you have to cut your calorie intake to a quarter of your daily calorie needs; you consume only 500 to 600 calories per day.

This plan allows you to choose whichever days of the week you prefer for fasting. You need to make sure there is one non-fasting day between. One typical pattern of following this plan is to make Monday and Thursday your fasting days, while the rest of the week will be non-fasting. Eat two to three small meals on every fasting day, then eat normally for the remainder of the week.

Again, eating "normally" does not mean you get to eat anything you want. You are discouraged from binge-eating junk foods as this can jeopardize your whole routine. You may gain weight instead of shedding it. Eat the same amount of food as you usually would if you weren't fasting at all.

If done the right way, the 5:2 diet can prove highly useful for weight loss. It helps you consume fewer calories per week, which enhances your body's metabolic rate. There is no definitive way to eat during the five-day fasting window. But there are approaches you can take.

For example, some people can't get their body moving without a small breakfast to jump-start the day. For others, starting the day with breakfast is a sure way to boost hunger throughout their day. People like that need to wait if they can before their first meal of the day.

Thus, this fasting method's meal plan may vary from person to person, although only slightly. On fast days, your schedules may include either of:

- Three small meals, which include an early breakfast, lunch, and late dinner
- Early afternoon meal and late-night dinner
- A brief breakfast and lunch, without dinner
- A single meal of breakfast or dinner

You can pick any of these schedules or change them from week to week. That decision is yours to make. The point is to drastically cut down the number of calories you consume. If you consume 1,800 calories on an average day, only consume 450 calories during your fasting window. If your daily calorie intake is usually 2,000, then reduce it to 500 calories on fast days.

If you do a lot of endurance exercise, don't fast on days when you work out. Consult with your doctor to make sure this fasting plan is compatible with any other physical activity you regularly engage in. Evaluate your training plan to make sure it aligns with the dieting plan.

Eat Stop Eat

This approach is one of the easiest you can take when it comes to intermittent fasting. As a beginner, if you cannot do the 12:12 method, you can begin your journey with this one. Brad Pilon, an intermittent fasting expert, is the originator of this method. Pilon researched short-term fasting and its benefits, and the findings were used to come up with the Eat Stop Eat fasting style.

According to Pilon, the best way to lose the extra pounds in your body is by fasting for 24 hours at least once or twice per week. During the non-fasting days, you can eat normally. But you are not to consume any calorie-containing food during your fasting window or days. By doing this, you can create a calorie deficit in your body, which will, over time, lead to effective weight loss.

For instance, if you typically consume 1800 calories daily, the Eat Stop Eat method two days a week will cause a calorie deficit of 3600 each week. To lose a pound of fat, you need a deficit of 3500 calories. Thus, you can potentially lose more than a pound every week if you follow this dieting style.

This method is not a fluke. A simple search on Google will bring up tons of positive reviews from people who have successfully used it to shed extra pounds. If done the right way, you can use Eat Stop Eat to lose up to 9 pounds in a month. That, of course, depends on your body, but using this approach will help you shed a couple of pounds.

As a newbie to the whole fasting thing, following this method is recommended because you do not have to fast every day. This means you don't have to worry about the fasting routine affecting your regular day-to-day schedule. You also have the freedom to decide when your fasting days are, which makes it easy to choose whenever is convenient for you.

For example, suppose weekend days allow you to engage in activities that can distract you from cravings. There, you can simply choose the weekend for your fasting window.

This diet is similar to the 5:2 plan, so many beginners confuse them, but there is a vital difference between both fasting styles. The 5:2 diet restricts your calorie intake on fasting days to 500. The Eat Stop Eat diet restricts you from calorie intake for 24 hours. During the fasting window, you may not consume any food or drink that contains calories.

Not eating for 24 hours might seem like a difficult task, and rightfully so. But with the 5:2 diet, the 500 calories intake can trigger hunger and facilitate physical discomfort. On the other hand, eating nothing within a 24-hour window helps suppress your appetite until your window elapses and ready for food consumption.

There is no specific drawback to using this style of fasting. But know that most of the scientific studies done on intermittent fasting have focused on the 16:8 and Alternate Day Fasting methods. Therefore, one cannot give science-backed evidence of any drawback.

Still, that does not imply that this approach is ineffective or has fewer advantages than other fasting methods. The only apparent drawback is that some people may find it difficult to fast for 24 hours without food intake. Consequentially, they may end up overeating when the eating window begins.

Any newbie to fasting is more likely to experience this slight problem. Nevertheless, once the body adapts to the new state of metabolism and energy balance, this problem will cease to exist. This fasting method is not appropriate for pregnant women, diabetics, or anyone with an eating disorder. Before you get started with Eat Stop Eat, learn your needs, goals, and fasting ability.

Alternate Day Fasting

Alternate day fasting (ADF) is relatively straightforward. It is an approach to intermittent fasting that involves fasting every other day. It has several versions of itself, but the end goal of all the versions is to help you cut down the intake of calories. One standard version of ADF is called modified fasting, which encourages you to consume 25% of your daily calorie intake on fasting days.

Basically, you fast on one day, eat what you want the next day, fast the following day again, and continue like that until you complete your fasting cycle. This way, you just need to limit what you eat half of the week. During the fasting window, you can consume as many calorie-devoid beverages and drinks as you desire.

The most common version of ADF is "The Every Other Day Diet." This version was popularized by Dr. Krista Vardy, who is also the researcher with the most studies done on ADF. Whether you consume the calories at lunch or dinner, the weight loss benefits remain the same. You may also consume small meals throughout the day if you don't go beyond the specified number of calories.

Depending on your body and needs, alternate-day fasting may prove easier for you than other types of intermittent fasting. A study on the effect of alternate-day fasting on weight loss among obese adults found this method is not necessarily superior to daily calorie restriction. Most of the ADF studies focus on the modified version, which allows you to consume 500 calories on fasting days. Some experts believe this is more sustainable than the full fasts.

It is impossible to pinpoint the specific effects of ADF on hunger. Depending on the individual, hunger may reduce on fasting days or remain unchanged. But the consensus is that calorie-restrictive fasting is much more convenient than full fasts.

All weight loss methods seem to trigger a drop in the body's resting metabolic rate. This happens when the body induces starvation mode. Technically, the process is called adaptive thermogenesis. It often occurs when an individual severely restricts their calorie intake.

When strict calorie restriction happens, the body automatically starts conserving energy by decreasing the calories it burns daily. This, inadvertently, causes weight loss to stop. Understandably, an experience like this can make you feel miserable. Fortunately, ADF does not appear to cause a dip in the body's metabolic rate, based on research.

Spontaneous Meal Skipping

This is an unstructured intermittent fasting plan that allows you to simply skip meals occasionally. For example, you may skip a meal when you don't feel hungry or don't have time to cook or eat.

There is a popular misconception that people have to eat every few hours to avoid losing muscle or going into starvation mode. Your body was designed to effectively handle prolonged hunger. So, missing a meal occasionally won't affect you in any way. It will help you lose or maintain your weight.

Thus, if you don't feel hungry on certain days, you can take advantage of that to skip breakfast or lunch and have a healthy dinner. Or, if you are traveling and can't get food anywhere, use that time to practice spontaneous meal skipping.

The method may not be as effective as other plans like 5:2 or 16:8, but it has its advantages. Just eat healthy meals during your eating window.

Warrior Diet

The warrior diet was created by Ori Hofmekler, an ex-member of the Israeli Special Forces, who became a fitness and nutrition expert. The diet is a type of intermittent fasting which is founded on ancient eating patterns followed by warriors. It involves eating very little during the day and then overeating at night.

Hofmekler says it is meant to "improve the way we eat, feel, perform, and look" by triggering stress in the body via reduced calorie intake. The result is to trigger the human "survival instincts."

This diet is not based on any science. It was designed purely on Hofmekler's personal beliefs and observations. To follow this diet, you have to under-eat for at least 20 hours of the day, then overeat as much food as you can at night.

During the fasting window, you are encouraged to eat vegetables, raw fruit, hard-boiled eggs, other dairy products in small amounts, and zero-calorie drinks. After the 20-hour window has passed, you can binge-eat whatever you want within the 4-hour eating window. But you are encouraged to stick to healthy, organic foods.

To start the warrior diet, you are urged to stick to a three-week plan segmented into different phases. The three-phase plan's basis is to enhance your body's ability to use fat as fuel or energy. The first phase in week one is for detox. Week two is called the "High fat" phase. The final phase is the "Concluding fat loss" stage.

Each phase encourages you to consume unprocessed, organic foods, but you still have the liberty of choosing what you eat. The last stage mostly cycles between the high carb and high protein intake. Once all three phases are completed, you are to begin all over again. But rather than go through the complete cycle, you may forgo the first two phases and simply adhere to the general guidelines.

The guidelines include consuming low-calorie foods and drinks for 20 hours and then consuming protein-rich, organic meals during your feasting phase.

The warrior diet has several limitations that make it inappropriate for most people. The 4-hour eating window makes it highly unsustainable for many people. It leaves little room for dieters to participate in regular social activities such as having lunch or breakfast with friends.

But this does not apply to everyone. Some people are not necessarily affected when they consume a few calories over the fasting period. You may experiment to determine if this pattern of eating is ideal for your lifestyle.

The warrior diet is inappropriate for any of the people below:

- Pregnant women
- Nursing mothers
- Children
- Athletes
- Those with eating disorders
- Underweight people
- Individuals with cancer, heart failure, type 1 diabetes, and other conditions

Some women may follow this diet with zero adverse effects. In contrast, others need to stay off it because of its impact on hormones. Common side effects include anxiety, insomnia, fluctuating periods, and other health disturbances.

Picking an intermittent fasting plan well suited to your lifestyle is crucial. You can experiment with a few strategies discussed to determine which is more appropriate for you. If you so wish, you can even change the pattern you use occasionally. Just don't do it too often.

As impressive as time-restricted eating is, it simply isn't for everyone. In the next chapter, you will discover if it is for you or not. Who can practice intermittent fasting and who can't? Let's learn more!

Chapter Four: Who Should and Who Should Not Fast

Fasting may be a useful weight-loss hack, but it certainly isn't for everyone. In pursuing health, intermittent fasting can be misused. Any diet that involves time-restricted eating for extended periods is most definitely not suitable for certain people. Several factors determine who should fast and who should not. It is best to know if fasting is safe for you before incorporating it into your daily routine.

If you are healthy and hydrated, fasting shouldn't be harmful to you. If you have health conditions, it may be bad for you. Typically, your body requires minerals, vitamins, and other nutrients to stay healthy.

Foods are your number one source of these nutritional requirements. Without getting enough, you could develop symptoms such as dizziness, fatigue, dehydration, and constipation. You may also find it difficult to withstand colder temperatures. For the wrong person, fasting can be life-threatening.

As long as you are healthy and fit with no diagnosed conditions that could jeopardize your health, you can fast. But if you have one or more of the following conditions, you shouldn't try intermittent fasting.

Diabetes

Diabetic individuals suffer frequent spikes and drops in their blood sugar levels throughout the day. The last thing they require is for fasting to heighten the fluctuation in their blood glucose responses.

Those with type 1 diabetes are especially cautioned to stay away from fasting because their pancreas cannot produce insulin, which is the hormone responsible for transferring sugar from the bloodstream to the body's different cells.

Individuals with type 1 diabetes need insulin injections to avoid inducing a state of hyperglycemia, which is when there is excess sugar in the bloodstream. If you are diabetic and on medication for insulin, you need to consult your doctor before intermittent fasting.

Fasting while you are on diabetes medications can cause a dangerous low in your blood sugar. But if your doctor gives the go-ahead, you will need close monitoring to continue with fasting. Anyone with low blood sugar should avoid intermittent fasting because consuming food every day is crucial to maintaining sufficient blood sugar levels.

Pregnancy or Breastfeeding

Fasting during pregnancy or while breastfeeding is a threat to child development. So, pregnant and breastfeeding women are not encouraged to engage in intermittent fasting because they have high caloric needs.

During pregnancy, a woman has to consume specific calories to aid milk production and fetal development. While no study has suggested that fasting can inhibit fetal growth, it is best to be on the safer side by fulfilling the daily calorie requirements. Fasting interferes with caloric intake, so the ideal thing is to stay away from it during pregnancy.

Even if you aren't pregnant, fasting may still not be ideal for anyone trying to get pregnant. Experts suggest that intermittent fasting may cause fertility issues and changes in menstruation due to hormonal effects. It also disrupts metabolism and may even prompt early menopause in women who are yet in their fifties.

Eating Disorders

The Academy of Nutrition and Dietetics says that disordered eating "is used to describe a range of irregular eating behaviors that may or may not warrant a diagnosis of a specific eating disorder."

Eating disorders are not described as a diagnosis. Instead, they are treated as a descriptive phase. Suppose one doesn't address irregular eating habits or patterns. In that case, it may turn into actual eating disorders such as bulimia nervosa, anorexia nervosa, or binge eating.

If you have ever experienced any irregular eating pattern or have an eating disorder, it is best to steer clear of intermittent fasting or any other type of fasting. Any diet that encourages restricting calorie intake can trigger a disorder in people with a history of irregular eating patterns. For everyone, but someone with a history, in particular, listening to your body is crucial.

You must be mindful of what makes you feel physical, mentally, and emotionally well. If time-restricted eating does not make you feel adequate, it means that intermittent fasting is not the right diet for you.

Sleep Problems

Getting enough sleep at night isn't a choice. Adequate sleep every night is a necessity. It is key to repairing and healing your muscles. Sleep supports brain function and maintains your emotional well-being.

Going to bed on an empty stomach can make it hard for your body to relax and sleep. Fasting makes the brain stay on alert, which inadvertently causes your body to be restless. If the end of your eating window is early in the day, falling asleep or staying asleep may become a struggle for you. Sleep inadequacy makes you vulnerable to a couple of health risks since sleep time is when your body can do all the healing and repairing work it is meant to do.

Additionally, blood sugar levels drop during the fasting window, and this can disrupt your sleeping pattern. You may wake abruptly during the night due to anxiety. A disrupted sleeping pattern is dangerous to your overall health. It is especially harmful if the disruption frequently happens during the most pivotal stage when the Random Eye Movement (REM) cycle occurs.

The REM stage is key to retaining vital information you learn and process during the day to commit it to memory. It happens multiple times throughout your sleep, which is why it is called a cycle. Besides these, disruptions can lead to other complications that may not immediately become apparent.

Not getting enough sleep can also interfere with weight management. If intermittent fasting causes you sleep problems, it might help you gain more weight instead of losing it.

Insufficient Muscle Mass

If you are trying to build your muscle mass, intermittent fasting may be unsafe for you. In fact, experts suggest that it is not ideal. Muscle building requires you to consume protein-rich foods several times throughout the day. This is better than jam-packing it in a single eating window.

Experts say this is because the average person's body cannot metabolize more than 35g of protein in a sitting. Suppose you want your body to metabolize properly. There, you are better off eating your protein meals at different times across your whole day. Without proper metabolization, excess protein stores as fat rather than muscle.

To build muscle, you need to spread your protein consumption through multiple meals in a day. Also, consume one protein-rich snack before bedtime. These are the two research-backed ways for you to achieve optimum muscle-building results. Narrowing your consumption window to just 8 or 12 hours is counteractive to this approach.

But if you would still like to go ahead, talk to your doctor about the safest ways to engage in intermittent fasting without countering your muscle-building effort.

Digestion Issues

Combining digestion problems with intermittent fasting can worsen their health situation. If you have any issue with digestion, you already know that they are cumbersome enough to deal with individually. Now, if you add an irregular eating schedule to the mix, you can compound the problem.

Extended periods of fasting can lead to more gastrointestinal distress. Even if you have no digestion problems, prolonged fasting can serve as a trigger. This happens because prolonged periods of fasting disrupt your digestive system's everyday activities. This results in indigestion, constipation, and bloating.

If you use an IF method that requires a prolonged fast, such as the warrior diet, you may consume one large meal at the end of your fasting window, but it can cause gastrointestinal stress. People with sensitive guts should be particularly wary of practicing any form of fasting.

Weak Immune System

Women who face a major illness or have just experienced one should not practice IF without seeking their doctor's advice first. Often, regular caloric intake is necessary to keep the immune system healthy and maintain lean muscle. It is even essential for those with a weak immune system or conditions such as cancer. It is something that you cannot compromise if you have any of both conditions.

Before you engage in fasting, speak to your doctor to make sure that your body can handle the effect. To boost your immune response, start by skipping IF from your dieting routine. There are tons of other dieting techniques safer for you to lose weight.

Besides these health reasons, many other factors may hinder your ability to fast effectively. Shown below are factors that hamper participation in intermittent fasting.

- **Lifestyle**

Intermittent fasting is not just a dieting technique; it is a lifestyle – and it must align or fit into the dieter's lifestyle. Your work schedule is part of what comprises your lifestyle. It influences your ability to make IF a part of your routine. If your work does not support the fasting hours, then there is little you can do.

For instance, if your job requires you to work the night shift, it may have a negative effect on you. Working the night shift means you sleep during the day. If you follow an IF technique with the eating window during the day, how do you work around that?

What if your fasting window falls within the time you are hard at work? Or worse, what if your schedule is inconsistent and prone to regular change? There, the fasting intervals can leave you feeling cold, give you headaches and mood swings. These side effects could make you less productive at work because they are distracting.

The ideal thing is to settle for another dieting strategy if intermittent fasting does not match your lifestyle.

- **Medications**

Some people are on medications with food as a prerequisite; in other words, their medications cannot be used in the absence of food. Without it, they can leave you feeling light-headed and nauseous, among many other side effects.

Prolonged fasting periods can also affect those who take supplements and vitamins daily. For example, those with anemia or low iron count in their bloodstream usually need to take iron supplements daily to maintain iron levels.

Iron supplements typically cause nausea, but the feeling can be suppressed with food. If you have a flexible schedule for taking your supplements, then fasting shouldn't be a problem, but if you have to take the medications at a specific time of the day with food, things may get a little tricky.

Ultimately, it is simply not ideal to start time-restricted eating if you are on medications that can't be administered without food intake.

• Job

Food provides energy and sustenance, which, in turn, enable you to focus. Extreme pangs of hunger make you think about food, diverting your attention from any tasks on the ground. Naturally, everyone reacts to periodic fasting differently. The side-effects generally depend on the individual doing the fasting.

In the initial stage, IF hinders everyone's ability to focus. If you have never had to go long periods without food, you will also experience this. If you have a job that requires intense focus and concentration, IF may pose a problem.

Although many people report energy increase during fasting windows, most people experience low energy levels, reduced concentration, and fatigue. These affect productivity. Suppose you have a career or regularly engage in activities that require great attention and energy. In that case, prolonged fasting may be impractical for you.

• Intensive Training

As you have likely assumed, combining intermittent fasting with any high-intensity activity or training cycle is not safe or ideal. You might practice intermittent fasting if you regularly engage in CrossFit or train for marathons. Usually, you will need to consume something tangible before exercising. This helps to power you through the duration of your workout.

It is also of extreme importance you eat something after you finish your workout. During an intense training exercise, you deplete your glycogen stores, and minor tears happen in your muscles. A recovery meal within two hours plus regular meals every four hours is the key to refilling our glycogen stores. It also helps to repair and rebuild the tears in your muscle throughout the rest of your day.

Skipping the post-training meal delays your recovery and eventually inhibits the build and repair of muscles, which is essential.

Whether you have any of the conditions explained above or not, you should still discuss intermittent fasting with your doctor before you begin. We all live in one big obesogenic food environment.

The U.S. is generally a toxic place because a significant percentage of the population does not engage in healthy eating habits. Even if nothing obstructs you from trying intermittent fasting, be sure that you have a robust social network to support you through your journey. This sometimes makes all the difference for dieters. With supportive friends and family members, enduring low-calorie days over the long haul should prove easy.

Chapter Five: How to Safely Lose Weight While Fasting

Losing weight after turning 50 involves more than simply fasting. You need more than diet and exercise. The key is not just to lose weight but to lose it healthily. Besides fasting, you must develop other habits crucial to boosting your overall health and wellness. These habits should be geared toward improving both your physical and mental health.

Even while fasting, there are steps you can take to shake up your whole routine. Incorporating new activities and habits into your daily schedule will enable you to lose weight healthily while improving your mental and physical wellness.

Below, you will find many of the best weight-loss habits according to expert fitness and wellness trainers and dietitians. Building up these habits and following any tips you learn in this chapter is your key to shedding pounds with intermittent fasting and ensuring they stay off your body for good.

Consult Your Doctor

The first step you should take as you begin your 50s' fitness journey is talking to your doctor. Discuss the weight loss plan you want to follow extensively to make sure it is practical for you.

Your doctor should assess your health's current state to inform you of any potential problems affecting your weight loss journey. More importantly, you should work together to create the perfect plan that includes diet, exercise, and other necessary things. If needed, your doctor may even recommend a personal trainer or physical therapist for you.

Some commonly used medications enable weight gain, so let your doctor check your prescription meds to evaluate if there are any. Trying to lose weight while on drugs that make that impossible is a futile exercise. Antidepressants, diabetes medication, and high blood pressure medications are common ones to look out for.

If you are on any of these, your healthcare provider should be able to replace them with weight-neutral medications that may even promote weight loss.

Set Realistic Weight Loss Goals

Being as realistic as possible is the key to healthy weight loss. Don't set out to lose 20 pounds in a month because not only is it unrealistic, but it is also unhealthy. Honesty is a virtue, so be honest with yourself about your needs and current state of health.

Consider how you feel. Are you as healthy as you should be? If you aren't, taking extreme weight loss measures should be last on your to-do list. Taking the step to lose weight is equal to making a huge life change, requiring mental fortitude.

You need to break down your goals into smaller, realistic ones. The more real they are, the more achievable. Focus on the little, positive changes that can make a difference in your lifestyle. Take your mind away from the number on the scale and concentrate on the things that matter. Doing that will give you the motivation you need to achieve all your goals.

The little achievements amount to the most prominent goals achieved. As the saying goes, "Triumph makes courage grow." So, the more you accomplish the small goals, the more your courage grows to make you push even further.

Do Hormone Checks

Things might get a little complicated here because most times, hormones aren't even responsible for weight gain. However, your physical examination with your doctor might show signs of hormone irregularities. If this happens, the right thing to do is to check on your hormone levels.

As you age, your body's hormone levels decline, making your body start storing fats instead of burning them. If the hormones are at abnormal levels, you may need to take steps to whip them back into shape.

This can go a long way toward helping you burn fat and lose weight. As a woman trying to get fit in your fifties, you must focus on your testosterone production. In the medical community, people tend to concentrate on the loss of estrogen in older women. Few people know testosterone sufficiency is just as important.

A study conducted at the University of Macau confirms that balance in testosterone levels promotes weight loss and shrinks belly fat by reducing blood glucose levels. So, getting your hormones checked is one way you can lose weight as healthily as possible.

Know Your Caloric Needs

Calorie needs in women vary depending on lean body mass, metabolism, size, and activity level. According to the Dietary Guidelines for Americans, the estimated caloric needs for women over 50 based on activity level are:

- Sedentary women: 1600 daily calories
- Moderately active women: 1800 daily calories
- Active women: 2000 to 2200 daily calories

These guidelines are for 50+ women who would like to maintain a healthy weight and remain fit. Knowing your daily calorie needs gives insight into the number of hours you can put into fasting weekly while giving your body what it needs. If you are active or moderately active and you plan to lose weight healthily, aim to consume about 1200 calories daily. This will help you lose up to 2 pounds per week.

Get Familiar with Your Numbers

Before you start any weight loss plan, calculate your body mass index (BMI) and use the scale at home to weigh yourself. Don't stop at that, though. Some other numbers affect your looks as you get older.

The first is your waist circumference. In some women, hormonal changes do not cause weight gain. Instead, they change the way they carry weight on their body. So, even when you aren't gaining weight, you may look like you are. Your waistline could become bigger, giving the appearance of weight gain. Most women notice weight gain in their mid-sections.

The second number to be familiar with is your body fat percentage. The older you get, the more likely it is that your body composition will change. A dip in your testosterone levels causes the loss of muscle mass, which changes body composition. So, even if your weight remains the same, you might look fatty due to muscle loss.

Evaluate Your Lifestyle

As you get older and closer to retirement, your interests naturally shift toward more leisurely activities. You may spend more time indulging yourself by entertaining friends, eating out in restaurants, reading, and generally practicing self-care. This is normal and understandable, but several of these activities may lead to weight gain if you aren't cautious.

To lose weight healthily, don't give up activities you enjoy, but making small changes and adjustments to your lifestyle can make all the difference. It can help alter your energy balance. For instance, if you like traveling, consider going on an active vacation rather than choosing a food-based cruise. If you enjoy cooking, spend your time in a healthy cooking class.

Eating in restaurants, entertaining friends, and increased travel could also mean you consume alcoholic beverages more frequently. Alcoholic calories add up more quickly than food calories, and they often add up in the mid-section. Additionally, it is difficult to make healthy food choices when you drink.

The bottom line is that you may need to eliminate alcohol from your diet or at least cut back on drinking if you want to reach your weight loss goals.

Get 8-Hours of Sleep Daily

Getting enough sleep is essential for people of all ages, but particularly for women over 50. Sleep helps regulate the hormones in charge of your appetite. It also enhances brain and cognitive function, prevents injury, and energizes you to stay active throughout the day.

Obese and overweight people get less sleep than those who do not fall into that category. When you regularly deprive yourself of sleep, your body automatically increases hormones such as cortisol and ghrelin. Respectively, these hormones increase hunger and stimulate the appetite.

Older women who get less than five hours of sleep every night are twice as likely to be overweight or obese as those who get a solid 7 to 8 hours of sleep a night. Therefore, having a consistent sleep schedule isn't only an excellent idea. It is a necessity for anyone looking to lose weight. Being consistent means you wake up and retire to bed around the same time every day. If you don't make this a habit, you stand the risk of becoming obese.

The CDC recommends 7 to 9 hours of sleep a night for women in their fifties.

Know Your Macronutrients

Three primary macronutrients are essential for healthy and effective weight loss after age 50. They are Carbohydrates, Protein, and Dietary Fat. Carb and protein give the body four calories per gram, while dietary fat provides nine calories per gram.

Based on the Institute of Medicine recommendations, women over 50 should get 45 to 65 percent of their daily calories from carbs, 10 to 35 percent from protein, and 20 to 35 percent from dietary fat.

Since protein and dietary fiber are known to promote satiety, which is necessary for weight loss, consider the following when consuming your daily 1200 calories:

- 40% of calories from carbs, which is 120g of carbs daily.

- 35% of calories from protein, which equals 105g of protein daily

- 25% of calories from dietary fat, which is 40g of fat daily

If you don't have the time to count macronutrient grams, try dividing your plate during mealtime. Doing that will make sure that you get your daily nutritional needs. It is an excellent way to properly portion your meals and get all the essential nutrients to stay optimally healthy while you are on the path to losing the extra pounds.

Increase Daily Physical Activities

Exercise and workouts are not the only ways to get active every day. You can increase the number of calories your body burns daily by getting certain activities done. This is a surefire way to promote weight loss or maintenance after age 50.

The following are a few activities and how many calories you'll burn in 30 minutes:

- Dancing: 112 calories
- Cooking: 93 calories
- Bowling: 112 calories
- Gardening: 167 calories
- House cleaning: 167 calories
- Horseback riding: 149 calories
- Weeding: 172 calories
- Painting: 186 calories
- Raking: 149 calories

The point is to avoid sitting down as much as you can throughout the day. Since you now know how many calories each activity can help burn, calculate how many calories you want to burn and put in the work. Even if you have to get a sit/stand desk at work, increase your physical activities.

Drink Plenty of Non-Calorie Drinks

Drinking plenty of water every day will prevent dehydration and reduce hunger. In the morning, try to drink up to four cups of water when you wake up. Do that before you consume your morning tea or coffee. Also, drink 2 cups of water before breakfast as this helps to boost satiety.

Several studies have shown that caffeine aids fat-burning and weight loss. It also improves mental alertness and provides the boost of energy you need to stay active throughout each day. To reap its fat loss benefits, try to drink at least 3 cups of coffee or tea each day—no need to fret because 500 mg of caffeine every day is considered safe for the average adult.

Balance Your Daily Workouts

Any exercise on a day-to-day basis is an excellent idea for most people. But in your fifties, you need to take a more balanced approach to workouts. In fact, having a balanced exercise and workout program is one of the most important things. With a balanced program, you can offset most hormonal changes and body composition issues that arise with aging.

You can work out however you deem fit, but any program you follow should contain the four elements below:

- **Strength Training** – Resistance training exercises aim to enhance muscle growth and development. Doing them will keep your metabolism healthy. Multiple studies have confirmed that strength training has age-related benefits for older people.

- **Flexibility Training** – This involves stretching exercises targeted at increasing your joints' motion range. Daily flexibility training will help you stay limber and comfortable as you juggle through your daily living activities.

- **Aerobic Training** – Daily cardiovascular activities regulate the decrease in metabolic rate, which comes with age. More importantly, they also help to improve heart health. Combined with intermittent fasting, they can help to manage heart health risks.

- **Stability Training** – Including functional training activities in your daily routine will help you maintain a stable, healthy, and youthful body and look. Stability exercises are fortunately simple and take minutes to perform. Daily workouts can help improve your posture, balance, and overall appearance.

More workouts and exercises will be discussed later in the book. In the section about exercise for women over 50, you will determine your workout routine's specific activities.

The ideal approach is to make a total of three changes as you include everything discussed here in your daily routine. Adding over three can make you feel overwhelmed, and you might even be tempted to end your weight loss journey.

Remember that everyone ages differently, so don't compare yourself to anyone else in your age group. Be kind to yourself as your body changes, but don't stop motivating yourself to stay smart and active and keep your body lean and healthy as you add more years to your age.

Mindful Eating

Mindfulness is a habit we must all cultivate. Mindful eating is one thing every dieter should have in their toolbox. Often, mindless eating results from stress. Improving your awareness of what you eat can help you manage your weight better.

Mindful eating is all about paying attention as you plan your meals and eat them. It helps you know how hungry or full you are to avoid overeating or under-eating. Using this technique means you leave your phone or newspaper when you eat. This fully immerses you in the present. By using the mindful eating technique, you can tell exactly how your foods taste. But the most important thing is that making mindful eating a way of life can make your weight loss goals more achievable.

The North Carolina State University conducted an online mindfulness-based weight-loss study which confirmed that individuals who practice mindfulness eating lost more weight on average than those in a standard food control group. This study was presented at the European Congress on Obesity.

Foods That Promote Healthy Weight Loss in Women Over 50

As crucial as mindful eating is to healthy weight loss, eating the right food is also essential. What you eat is just as important as when you eat and what you do when eating. As you grow older, your body requires more specific foods and vitamins. It is usual for nutritional needs to change over different phases in life.

In youth, your nutritional requirements are geared toward growth and maintaining your body for procreation, should that be a goal for you. After age 50, they become targeted at keeping your mind and body in an optimal state of health. This, of course, includes leaving the extra fat off and looking as fit as possible.

Maintaining optimal health depends on what you eat. As you age, what you eat becomes more important than ever. Remember that your metabolic rate drops when you reach the 50-years mark. You need to consume foods that your body will find easier to break down and convert to fuel instead of adding them to the fat storage.

And some vitamins become more vital to protect you against diseases and general or specific health issues. Thus, you are responsible for making sure the foods you consume the most contain those essential vitamins that your body requires to stay healthy.

Shown below are foods that should be a part of your diet to keep your mind sharp and your body strong as you get rid of unwanted fat storage.

• Fiber-Rich Foods

You have likely learned the importance of fiber-rich foods from experience, as most people do. Gastrointestinal function declines in older people. Due to this, you must focus on consuming sufficient fiber to keep the system running smoothly.

Not only does fiber aid gastrointestinal function operate without hiccups, but it also reduces inflammation and cholesterol. It does all this while ensuring a release of energy-filled carbs into your bloodstream.

Ensure that you eat as much as 30g of fiber daily to keep your system going at a healthy pace. Raspberries, lentils, whole-wheat pasta, and green peas are a few of the richest fiber sources.

• B12 Foods

Stomach acidity decreases as the body ages. Getting enough B12 vitamins in your diet becomes harder. Stomach acid aids the release of B12 from the foods you eat to maintain your nervous system's health. This also helps critical metabolic processes.

Over the age of 50, approximately 10-30% of women experience difficulty absorbing the B12 from their foods. Those who are on medications that suppress stomach acid especially find it harder to get B12 from goods. On average, you should get up to 2.4 micrograms of this essential vitamin per day.

Dairy and foods from animals, such as meat, seafood, and egg, contain high amounts of vitamin B12. But you can also get it from your whole-grain cereals and other B12-fortified foods. If you have reason to believe that you are not getting adequate B12, discuss your concerns with your doctor, and they will probably recommend a B12 supplement or multivitamin to include in your diet.

- **Potassium-Rich Foods**

Bananas are probably the most popular source of potassium. It is commonly known that the risk of heart disease and stroke increases with age. An excellent way to lower the risk is to consume foods that are excellent sources of potassium. Examples include bananas and avocados.

The World Health Organization suggests that potassium can play a pivotal role in lowering the risks associated with blood pressure. The recommendation from the WHO says that women over 50 should consume a daily 4700 mg of potassium.

Besides bananas or avocados, potatoes and pistachios are also good sources of potassium. One potato contains around 900 mg of potassium. A cup of pistachios contains 1200 mg, an avocado has over 700 mg per cup, and a single banana has 400 mg.

- **Calcium-Rich Foods**

Calcium is recognized as the number one go-to nutrient for anyone looking to build and maintain strong bones and teeth. But most people don't know that it is key to the heart's function. Not only that, but it also helps make sure that the muscles and nervous system function as efficiently as they should.

The goal is for any woman over 50 to consume at least 1200 mg of calcium every day. But intake may sometimes be an issue due to two things. The first is that lactose-intolerant people may have a problem getting enough calcium, especially as they age. The second thing is that insufficient vitamin D in the body makes it hard to absorb calcium. Note that vitamin D also helps to boost immune function.

Scientific research has shown that as a person ages, access to vitamin D through sunlight and other fatty foods, added to the inability to absorb vitamins as efficiently as before, results in significantly below-standard levels of this essential vitamin.

The key to combatting these two problems is to consume more leafy greens such as kale, mustard, collards, and bok choy. You may also add sardines and canned salmon and tofu made with a calcium compound to your diet.

You may also need to ask your doctor to check your vitamin D level to know if you are getting enough vitamins. The consensus is that women should be within 70 nmol/L. If you don't have enough vitamin D, try getting at least 15 minutes of sunlight every day. Also, take any supplement recommendations from your doctor.

• **Turmeric and Cinnamon**

One other thing changes as you get older – taste. With age comes a decline in the production of saliva and your ability to perceive taste. To avoid losing that ability completely, consider experimenting with spices such as turmeric.

Research has shown that turmeric boosts immune function and reduces inflammation in the joints, preventing arthritis in older women. The main compound in turmeric is curcumin, which scientific studies suggest may have an authentic effect on certain forms of cancer and even Alzheimer's.

Cinnamon is another spice that should go into your cooking rotation. It is recognized as a potent anti-inflammatory and anti-microbial agent. It also helps regulate blood sugar levels by slowing the rate at which the tummy empties after meals. You may also use cinnamon therapeutically to manage your body's sensitivity to type 2 diabetes.

Besides making these important foods a part of your cooking plan for your eating windows, also follow these general guidelines for healthy eating. Sticking to them will help in your quest to lose weight healthily.

• Reduce saturated fats from your diet. Doing that will decrease the risk of cardiovascular disease. Eat more healthy fats derived from lean meats, low-fat dairy, fish, olive oil, nuts, and plant-based foods like avocado.

• Minimize or eliminate processed foods and drinks from your diet. Some of these include cookies, candies, chips, cakes, and pastries. Refined foods are known to increase inflammation in the body, leading to an increased risk of diabetes, cancer, and heart disease.

Follow every tip discussed. You can fast, lose weight, and stay fit, all while maintaining desirable physical and mental health.

Chapter Six: Hormones and Weight Loss

Hormones are chemicals secreted in the endocrine system by the glands. They travel through the bloodstream to your tissue and organs, telling them what to do and when to do it. They are crucial to regulating most of the primary bodily functions and processes, and they have an undeniable impact on your overall functioning.

Hormones do their jobs well when they are in a balanced state. But sometimes, they can become too much or too little in the bloodstream. This is when hormonal imbalance occurs. Due to the vital role hormones play in the body, a slight imbalance in hormonal secretion can trigger a ripple effect throughout your body.

Hormonal imbalance is one of the leading causes of weight gain in women over age 50. Add it to other factors that come with menopause, and weight loss becomes an almost unachievable goal for older women. Unexplained weight gain or weight loss (depending on whether the hormone is oversecreted or under-secreted) is the leading sign of imbalanced hormones.

Everyone experiences naturally driven periods of imbalance in hormone production. Fluctuations typically occur at different points in life. Sometimes, improper functioning of the endocrine system causes imbalance.

There are different endocrinal glands across the body, and they are all responsible for other organs. Some include:

- Adrenal glands
- Hypothalamus glands
- Thyroid and parathyroid glands
- Pituitary glands
- Pineal gland
- Gonads
- Pancreatic islets

Varying medical conditions can affect some of these endocrinal glands. Lifestyle habits and certain environmental factors may also play a role in hormonal imbalance, but sometimes, it just happens with age.

Many changes you experience between 40 and 50, such as menopause and decreased metabolism, are caused by a decline in hormone production. This naturally happens with age and has a significant impact on weight gain or loss. Increased hunger due to the overdrive in appetite hormones is a common symptom of a hormonal condition.

Sometimes, weight gain in your older age has nothing to do with eating habits or exercise routines. For most women over 50, misfiring hormones are the leading reason behind the unwanted pounds adding up.

To lose weight, you have to harmonize your hormone levels, and this requires focusing on more than one hormone. Interestingly, many people assume that estrogen is the only hormone that matters when managing weight issues in menopausal age, but it is far from the fact.

But first, how can you be sure that your hormones are responsible for the new extra weight? There are signs to watch out for. Getting familiar with these signs can help you identify the exact cause of weight gain so you can work on a targeted solution.

- **Bigger Waistline While Eating Right**

Suppose love handles suddenly appear around your waist even though you've had a reasonably flat tummy for the majority of your life. This is the number one sign that hormonal imbalance is at work. As you age, your body becomes more resistant to insulin. That drives it to store instead of burning fat.

Also, your estrogen becomes more dominant as you enter your perimenopause stage and beyond, leading to even more insulin resistance. All these cause your belly fat to build up and your waist to become bigger.

- **Your Sugar Craving Increases**

Insulin resistance can increase diabetes risk, but that is not all it does. It also affects other vital hormones. For instance, insulin resistance affects leptin, the hormone that lets your body know when your stomach is full—the higher your insulin resistance, the more your leptin levels increase.

Increased leptin, regardless of what you think, does not make you put down the spoon and stop eating. Instead, it results in dysfunctional leptin receptors. When not functioning correctly, the receptors stop alerting your brain when you are full. Due to that, you do the direct opposite of what your leptin is designed to regulate. In other words, you continue eating because your brain does not send the signal to stop.

- **Frequent Mood Swings**

As you reach the perimenopausal age and eventually the post-menopausal age, estrogen levels start fluctuating frequently. The results of this are mood swings and weight gain in your belly. It explains why women are more susceptible to mood disorders than men.

A study conducted by the University of Wisconsin on the Neurobiological Underpinnings of the Estrogen found that women's estrogen levels fluctuate more frequently during menopausal transitions and reproductive cycle events. This also tends to be the time when women report depression and recurrent depression the most.

Estrogen levels naturally fluctuate during menopause, leading to mood swings and weight gain. More light will be shed on this later in this chapter.

• Never-Ending Stress

If you find you are always stressed, that means your cortisol hormone is on overdrive. As you might know, cortisol is also called the stress hormone. It often increases when your body senses overwhelming anxiety and may cause stubborn weight gain, particularly in your midsection.

When you experience high levels of stress and anxiety, your body triggers the fight-or-flight response, which you may call the "survival mode." Cortisol production increases when this happens, and your body receives signals to do more storing and less burning of fat.

• Exhaustion Without Sleep

Exhaustion and insomnia are possible signs that hormones are responsible for your weight gain. So, look out for them. Not getting adequate sleep can cause fatigue, which results in stress-induced insomnia. All of these affect your hormone production, especially cortisol levels.

Increased cortisol production causes thyroid production to decrease, which leads to central weight gain. It can also affect the hormones in charge of muscle growth, tissue building, and overall health.

To help you better understand how much effect your hormones can have on weight gain and weight loss, more specific insight will be provided on each hormone mentioned so far and others and how they influence fat storage in the body.

At least five hormones experience imbalance and affect your ability to metabolize appropriately once you reach menopause. Together, they sabotage your weight loss efforts and make you believe that you can no longer get rid of extra fats. These five hormones are:

- Estrogen
- Cortisol
- Thyroid
- Testosterone
- Insulin

One by one, let's delve deeper into these hormones and how they can influence your weight loss journey as a woman trying to burn fat and stay fit in your fifties.

Estrogen

When you hear the word "estrogen," you probably think of a single hormone. Contrary to most people's beliefs, estrogen consists of three major hormones – estriol, estradiol, and osteon.

Estrogen is one of the primary sex hormones in females, but men also secrete it, although in smaller amounts. Declining estrogen levels affect men's waistlines just as they affect women's waistlines in later years.

Women naturally produce higher amounts of estrogen, which shapes their unique hourglass figure. But with age, estrogen levels decrease, causing women to assume a more masculine shape and figure.

Estrogen is also one hormone that causes women challenges in the fat department as they get older. Out-of-balance estrogen levels can turn the average woman into a fat-storing machine. This sometimes happens rapidly, leaving a woman feeling frustrated and confused.

Estrogen does not work alone. It operates in tandem with a group of steroid hormones known as progesterone. Your progesterone levels also decline with age. The symptoms typically include breast swelling, mood swings, trouble sleeping, irritability, and water retention.

If you have the coveted hourglass shape, that is courtesy of estrogen. This hormone is in charge of storing and regulating fat in the hips and things. When working together, progesterone and estrogen stop the body from storing fat around the waist, providing that tiny waist women like to flaunt. Still, the harmonious relationship between both sometimes suffers interference.

Stress affects the progesterone's function, leading to weight gain in and around the belly. The fat here is usually difficult to shift because progesterone levels are lower than estrogen levels in most women.

High levels of stress and anxiety negatively impact the production of progesterone. So, when you notice fat accumulating around your waist area without you increasing your calorie intake or reducing physical activity, that is a sign you need to cut down on the stress-inducing events in your day-to-day life. Doing that will help keep progesterone levels balanced.

Since estrogen production decline rarely happens until later in life, women believe that excess estrogen is a good thing. Unfortunately, that is not the case. Estrogen dominance can lead to excessive weight gain when progesterone isn't at the same levels.

When your body produces too much estrogen, you cannot reap the positive effects of progesterone. This is because the overproduction of estrogen leads to overstimulation of the brain and body.

The confusion around estrogen-progesterone partnership arises when you find that your estrogen levels are low, but you are estrogen-dominant anyway. Dominance occurs when an estrogen to progesterone ratio is higher than usual. That means you need more progesterone to keep estrogen levels from acting erratically.

How do you know when you are estrogen-dominant in your fifties?

- Weight gain in the abdomen and hips area
- Inability to lose weight easily
- Bloating
- Water retention
- Mood swings
- Slow metabolism
- Fatigue
- Trouble sleeping

If you notice that your weight gain isn't responding to dietary changes or workout routines, below is a quick quiz you can take to check if estrogen is dominating progesterone in an imbalanced way.

Do you sweat a lot at night?

o Yes, every night

o Once a week

o 3 to 5 times a week

o Never

Do you have hot flushes?

o Once a day

o 5 times a day or more

o 1 to 5 times a day

o Never

Have you gained a lot of weight recently?

o Yes

o No

Do you experience abnormal periods?

o Yes

o No

o Used to experience abnormal periods but no longer have periods

Do you suffer from low libido?

o Yes

o No

Do you experience bloating?

o Yes

o No

o Occasionally

Do you have food cravings?

o Yes

o No

o Sometimes

Your answers to these questions will help you determine whether you have estrogen dominance based on what you have learned about its symptoms. Eventually, you will discover how intermittent fasting can help you manage hormonal imbalances to promote healthy weight loss. But meanwhile, let's move on to the next hormone that affects weight gain and loss.

Cortisol

So far, you know how cortisol affects weight loss, but let's go deeper to explore the relationship between both. Earlier, you learned that cortisol is the body's stress hormone. Its production increases when the body activates the survival mode, otherwise known as the fight or flight response.

Elevated stress causes an imbalance in your cortisol, adrenaline, and DHEA hormones. High-stress levels stimulate your adrenal glands, helping to excessively produce all these hormones. When the stress levels drop, hormones should naturally balance out. However, occasionally, the hormones remain irregular for prolonged periods, causing a ripple of adverse effects on your body. That, unfortunately, includes weight gain.

Of all these hormones, cortisol has the strongest link with weight fluctuation in older women. Excess or deficiency of the hormone can affect your thyroid functions and blood sugar levels, which triggers signs of slow metabolism and weight fluctuation.

The major stressors that may contribute to cortisol imbalance are:

- Inadequate sleep
- Emotional imbalances
- Excessive carb intake
- Inconsistent work schedule
- Frequent delay of meals
- Toxin exposure

Cortisol has an exciting and vital relationship with insulin, which controls your blood sugar levels. An increase in cortisol levels promotes insulin resistance, which causes blood sugar levels to suffer instability. This typically leads to weight gain, higher blood sugar and increases the risk of type 2 diabetes.

On the other hand, cortisol levels can also dramatically decrease. This is known as adrenal exhaustion. When it happens, blood sugar levels decline, resulting in hypoglycemia. This condition is linked to unhealthy weight loss and decreased stress tolerance.

Increased or decreased imbalance in cortisol levels can cause metabolism to decline, particularly in women over 50. To a significant extent, cortisol levels are also responsible for the optimal production of hormones in the thyroid gland.

When the thyroid gland functions correctly, it helps to maintain a healthy metabolism, regardless of age. But imbalanced cortisol levels can potentially impair the body's ability to convert inactive thyroid to its active form. Again, this can lead to a decreased thyroid problem, leading to low metabolism and unwanted weight gain.

To address the hormonal imbalance that concerns your cortisol and thyroid, you may need to consult your doctor, who will advise you on the best steps to identify the exact issue responsible for low metabolism and weight gain.

After this, you can work with your doctor to discuss diet recommendations, which could be intermittent fasting, plus other lifestyle changes and the introduction of nutritional supplements to your daily routine.

Thyroid

The thyroid gland is one of the glands in your endocrine system. Its job is to produce the thyroid hormones, which go into your bloodstream and transmit to your tissues and organs to help your body put energy to use. The point of this is to help the brain, heart, muscles, and several other organs function as efficiently as they should keep your body running without hitches. So, thyroid hormones are quite important. Now, what is the nature of the relationship between thyroid hormones and weight?

Medical experts have affirmed an intricate relationship between thyroid disease, metabolism, and body weight for a long time. Thyroid hormones regulate metabolism. You can determine your metabolism by measuring the amount of oxygen your body uses over a specific timeframe.

This measurement, if made at rest, is called the basal metabolic rate (BMR). The BMR is one of the earliest ways of assessing thyroid status in patients. Those with nonfunctioning thyroid glands were discovered to have low BMRs, and those with overactive thyroid glands had higher BMRs.

Later, advanced research linked the initial observations with the measurements of thyroid hormone levels. They found that low thyroid levels were associated with low BMRs, and high thyroid levels were connected with high BMRs. The BMR measurement isn't used as much nowadays due to the test's complexity. Still, it does establish a link between weight and thyroid state.

People with hyperthyroidism, which is when the thyroid glands are overactive, have elevated BMRs. Those with overactive thyroid hormones experience weight loss, which can be extreme in some cases. Furthermore, weight loss is influenced by the extent of the thyroid's overactivity.

This means that when the thyroid becomes hyperactive, the BMR increases, meaning that a person has to consume more calories to maintain their body weight. If the number of calories isn't increased to match the excess calories burned, it will cause extreme weight loss.

As indicated before, the factors that regulate appetite, activity, and metabolism are complex. At the center of this complex system is the thyroid hormone. But on average, the more severe hyperthyroidism is, the more extreme the weight loss is.

Hyperthyroidism is an abnormal state, which is why it promotes unhealthy weight loss. Suppose you are losing weight in your 50s, even without dieting or anything. There, the right thing to do is to check for any possible imbalance in your thyroid hormones.

Naturally, any weight loss caused by an overactive thyroid will eventually go away when you treat and reverse the condition. However, this is tricky. If you continue eating more calories, it can cause excess weight gain.

On the other hand, hypothyroidism – which refers to underactive thyroid gland activity, has a relationship with weight gain. BMR is typically lower in people with underactive thyroid hormones, which lead to weight gain.

The amount of weight gained often depends on the severity of hypothyroidism. But the decline in BMR due to underactive thyroid is much less extreme than the increase experienced in hyperthyroidism. This leads to more slight alterations in weight.

The exact cause of weight gain in hypothyroid people is tricky. It sometimes has nothing to do with calorie or fat accumulation. Most times, the excess weight happens due to the accumulation of water and salt. Rarely does massive weight gain happen due to hypothyroidism.

Generally, most people don't gain more than ten pounds of fat due to the thyroid, depending on the gland's level of inactivity. If weight gain is the only present sign of hypothyroidism, your weight gain likely has little to do with the thyroid.

Thyroid hormones have been used as a tool for healthy weight loss. Increasing thyroid hormone to elevate the hormone levels may not cause a dramatic weight change. But thyroid hormone treatment can help achieve more weight loss than some dieting plans. Naturally, you have to talk with your doctor to determine if you need the treatment. However, fasting can help you achieve balance in production to avoid gaining unwanted excess weight.

Testosterone

Testosterone may be the primary sex hormone in men, but it is present abundantly in women too. It may not be as much, but it certainly plays some vital role, particularly for losing fat.

This hormone is responsible for muscle growth in both men and women. Testosterone deficiency automatically makes you predisposed to excessive fat storage. To understand and manage testosterone imbalance, it's essential to understand its role in weight gain and fat loss.

One crucial function of this hormone is to build and maintain muscle mass and promote muscle growth. It also boosts bone strength. Your hormonal levels decline as you add years, which is why muscle and bone loss occurs the older you get.

Just as it promotes muscle growth, testosterone also suppresses fat gain. So, when the levels decline, its fat-suppressing ability declines as well. As a result, you may start gaining more fat than you want.

As explained earlier, muscles use way more calories than fat tissue. With the loss of muscle in older women, you are at the risk of overeating and storing extra calories as body fat. This means that reduced muscle mass due to testosterone decline or deficiency is the primary reason older women start gaining extra pounds with age.

Here's where it gets interesting – obesity may suppress testosterone levels in older women. Multiple studies have shown that obese women have lower testosterone levels than normal-weight ones. Therefore, excessive fat storage in the body may suppress your testosterone levels.

The key to preventing weight gain due to low testosterone levels is to work on increasing them naturally. The number one sign of decline in older women is reduced muscle mass. So, if you lose muscles at an alarming rate, your testosterone might be dangerously low. There,

there are natural steps you can take to drive the levels up to aid weight loss.

A few include:

- Getting enough vitamin D
- Eating zinc-rich foods
- Getting adequate sleep
- Minimizing the stressors in your daily life and environment
- Strength training

When you combine these with intermittent fasting and other effective weight loss techniques, these steps will get your testosterone levels back up so you can lose weight without worries.

The right thing to do if you suspect you have testosterone deficiency is to reach out to your doctor. A simple blood test will reveal the truth, and your doctor will tell you the next step. He or she may recommend testosterone replacement therapy, which is frankly the best way to stabilize your hormonal levels. But this should only be a resort if the natural methods do not work for you.

Insulin

Insulin and weight gain usually go hand in hand. The more insulin your body produces, the more likely you are to add extra pounds. Still, weight control or loss is not entirely impossible. You have only to normalize your insulin levels to reduce or avoid weight gain.

Insulin is much misunderstood. Too little insulin in the bloodstream can cause serious health problems, and too much can cause weight gain. A general side effect for those who take insulin is weight gain.

Therefore, if you have any condition that requires you to take insulin, you are more prone to weight gain. Add that to age-triggered weight gain, and you realize that you have a lot to do if you want to lose weight effectively.

How does insulin contribute to weight gain?

When you take insulin, glucose enters your cells, making your blood glucose levels drop. That is how insulin treatment is supposed to work. But consider you consume more calories than you need to achieve a healthy weight, depending on your activity level. In that case, your cells might end up getting more glucose than necessary. This means that they can't use it all. Glucose not used by the cells eventually stores as fat in the body.

Note that insulin does not precisely stop your body from burning fat. But it does have a significant influence on the rate at which fat burns. That is because, apart from insulin being the body's blood glucose regulator, it also:

- **Inhibits Lipolysis**

Throughout lipolysis, accumulated fatty acids move out of your fat cells into the bloodstream, where they are used for energy. When insulin levels are high, it inhibits this process by blocking the release of fatty acids, thus ensuring that you get fewer fatty acids to fuel your metabolically active tissues. Due to this, your body's ability to burn fat is significantly reduced.

- **Initiates Lipogenesis**

Lipogenesis is when fatty acids move from your bloodstream into your fat cells, where they are stored away for later use. Many people call this the "fat storage mode," and they try as much as possible to avoid it.

Besides, lipogenesis can cause carbohydrates to convert and store as fat. This process is called Novo lipogenesis. Novo lipogenesis only happens when there is a surplus of carbs and calories, usually in meaningful amounts. You consistently burn fewer calories than you eat. As a result, insulin can sometimes be a strong villain in your quest to burn and lose fat.

The key is to keep your insulin as low as possible to lose weight healthily. Without doing that, you might keep adding extra pounds. Eating fewer calories can help you keep your insulin levels down. That is why intermittent fasting is such an ideal dieting strategy for weight loss.

If done the right way, intermittent fasting can help you manage most hormonal imbalances responsible for weight gain in your older age. It increases insulin resistance. Doing that helps your cells recognize insulin more effectively, tapping into the fat-burning mechanism that allows natural weight loss.

Fasting increases the growth hormone, one of the crucial hormones your body needs to burn fat and increase muscle mass. You can't immediately detect your growth hormone levels when you eat. If you always eat and snack from daybreak until you retire to bed, you aren't giving your growth hormone the breather it needs to repair your muscle mass. On the other hand, Fasting can help minimize the rate at which you eat, causing your hormone to increase by up to 2000 percent.

Finally, intermittent fasting decreases cortisol levels and increases melatonin. Cortisol is the stress hormone, while melatonin is the sleep hormone. A balance in your cortisol and melatonin levels can be achieved with intermittent fasting and a proper workout routine. You need balanced melatonin to sleep and rest. When your melatonin levels are stabilized, you don't have to worry about insomnia and not getting enough sleep.

High levels of the sleep hormone make you feel dizzy and tired, so you can rest until the morning. Then, cortisol gives the mental awareness and energy you require to get the day going after you wake.

And when you are well-rested, other hormones responsible for weight loss and weight gain are positively affected. So, using intermittent fasting to balance your cortisol and melatonin is a win-win situation.

Homeostasis is vital for good health and wellness. It is your key to feeling and looking good. Paired with proper nutrients and a healthy workout program, intermittent fasting can help you achieve homeostasis to promote weight loss even as you get older.

Intermittent fasting is just one way of balancing your hormones. Besides this, there are other things you can do. You can redefine your diet and make sure it is filled with food that regulates and balances your hormone levels.

- **Carbs:** Don't stop eating carbs because you believe they contribute to weight gain. Well, you may stop eating carbs, but only the bad ones. Add more "good" carbs to your diet. Examples of good carbs include unprocessed whole grains, beans, vegetables, and fruit.

- **Organic:** Be more organic with your food choices to keep your hormones balanced. Organic foods and drinks are typically devoid of growth hormones. Also, it is believed that pesticides contribute to hormonal disruption in older and younger women. Add more root vegetables and leafy greens to your diet as they give your body the complex carbs it needs.

- **Kale:** Eating kale is excellent, but too much of it can disrupt your hormones. It is best to consume cruciferous vegetables as moderately you can. Kale contains goitrogens, which can block iodine from entering your thyroid gland. Your body requires iodine to secret the thyroid hormones, which are necessary for normal metabolism. More dairy in your diet can help you get enough iodine into your thyroid gland. But this doesn't mean you should skip out on kale totally. You can still eat it, but don't make it too much.

• **Probiotics and Prebiotics:** Gut health is crucial to hormonal balance. Unbalanced hormones affect your microbiome and gut barrier. This can cause inflammation issues. Add more probiotics food like yogurt, sauerkraut, and fermented foods to your diet. Also, prebiotics such as asparagus, bananas, and shiitake mushrooms should be a constant. All of these will keep your hormones balanced and your guts healthy.

• **Healthy Fats:** The AARP recommends that consuming more healthy fats such as olive oil, coconut oil, avocados, and sweet potatoes can help maintain estrogen levels balanced in the body. So, add more of these to your diet as well.

To wrap it up, ensure you eat less sugar, gluten, dairy, etc. You don't have to get rid of them. Just limit your consumption of them, as overeating can spike your insulin levels and disrupt other hormones crucial to keeping fit.

Hormones have a massive impact on the body's functioning. However, they decline with age, then affecting what they impact. To keep your body and mind healthy and sound, your hormones have to be balanced.

Imbalance in hormones can lead to many issues, including weight gain. That is precisely why you should be familiar with them and learn how you can manage hormonal imbalance to achieve your weight loss goals, regardless of aging.

Chapter Seven: The First Days of Intermittent Fasting

Getting started with intermittent fasting can be arduous if you have never gone hungry for a prolonged period. The very idea is daunting. It's normal for people to think, "Oh, I can't do this. I won't last the day. I give up" before fasting at all. But these negative thoughts will be much less prominent in your head when you know what to expect.

What are the first few days of intermittent fasting like? How long does it take your body to acclimatize with the new routine? What are the side-effects you might experience when you start fasting? The answers to these and many other questions will give you an insight into what to expect as you begin periodic fasting.

First, do not see intermittent fasting as a duty or task you owe your health and body. That just takes the fun out of everything. Instead, consider it a self-experiment – something you are doing to get to know more about your body and what makes it tick.

Break down your plan into small, doable actions that can be achieved step-by-step. That way, you can be guaranteed to finish with the program. As the fasting days go by, ensure you observe, analyze, and put down what you discover about your body and intermittent fasting. At the end of the fasting period, make your conclusion as to whether intermittent fasting is right for you.

Doing it that way makes it less of something to commit to and more of something to learn about. So, it doesn't feel like a task you have to endure. Instead, it feels like a process you are gaining knowledge from. This method makes it easy for you to start and finish your intermittent fasting plan. As humans, we learn best by doing.

There are different fasting stages, and they all have various hallmark features, as you will notice when you begin. What does each entail?

Fed State

The fed state is the first stage of fasting, and it is initiated within the early few hours after your eating window. It occurs as your body digests and breaks down nutrients from food for absorption. During this stage, your blood sugar levels rise, and your body secretes high amounts of insulin.

The insulin level in your bloodstream depends on your meal's composition, the number of carbs you ate, and your body's sensitivity to insulin. Extra glucose is stored in muscles and the liver as glycogen. Meanwhile, the levels of leptin and ghrelin also change. Ghrelin levels decrease because you have just eaten. Remember that ghrelin stimulates hunger. Leptin, on the other hand, increases to suppress your appetite.

Remember that the stages in IF occur in a cycle. The fed-fast state resets back to the fed state if you consume food during the fasting window. This makes it impossible for your body to complete the whole cycle. Also, the provided state's duration depends on the composition and size of the meal you consumed.

Early Fasting State

Three to four hours after you eat, your body shifts into the early fasting state. This stage lasts until about 18 hours. In this phase, your insulin and blood sugar levels begin to decrease, pushing your body to start converting stored carbs (glycogen) into sugar to use as fuel.

As this phase nears its end, you will eventually run out of glycogen stores, and your body will start the search for another energy source. This heightens lipolysis, which is a process in which your body breaks down fat cells into smaller molecules so they can serve as an alternative energy source. At the same time, your body converts amino acids into energy.

Most of the intermittent fasting plans explained in chapter three-cycle are between the first stage (fed state) and the second stage (early fasting state).

Fasting State

To enter the fasting state, you must have fasted from around 18 hours to 2 days. So, if you fast today and skip fasting the next day, your body might not trigger the fasting state. By this stage, your body has completely depleted the glycogen stores and has broken down fat stores and protein for fuel.

The result is that your body produces ketone bodies – compounds produced when fat is converted into fuel. Your body goes into ketosis, which is a metabolic state where your body turns to fat as its primary energy source. But you might not transit into ketosis when you enter the fasting state. It sometimes happens later on.

As with the early fasting state, your last meal's size and composition determine how quickly your body transitions into ketosis. Individual differences may also play a part.

Common signs of ketosis include:

- Fatigue
- Fruity smelling breath
- Decreased appetite
- Weight loss
- A higher number of ketone bodies in your breath, blood, or urine,

Ketosis is the main result those who follow the ketogenic diet aim to achieve. By getting the body to reach ketosis, weight loss is achieved.

Note that shorter forms of intermittent fasting may not reach ketosis unless you follow a low-carb diet. By decreasing your carb intake, your body can quickly run out of glycogen and use fat as its primary fuel source.

Starvation State

You may also call this the long-term fasting state. After extended fasting periods, your body initiates this phase. It typically occurs around 48 hours after eating. In this state, insulin and blood sugar levels continue to drop, and beta-hydroxybutyrate (BHB) levels steadily rise. BHB is a type of ketone body.

In this same phase, your kidneys activate gluconeogenesis and generate sugar via this process. This serves as the primary fuel source for the brain. Ketone bodies also provide energy for your brain. The processing of branched-chain amino acids (BCAAS), some of the essential amino acids, is steadily reduced to conserve muscle tissue in the body. Understand that you shouldn't do long-term fasts unless your medical doctor gives the go-ahead.

These are the four phases you go through during intermittent fasting. Depending on the number of hours you fast, you may not reach some of these states in the fed-fast cycle.

Each phase changes the primary energy source for your body and hormones that concern metabolism.

How to Practice Fasting Safely

Unless you do it properly, fasting can pose a danger to your health. That is why you should know the right tips to follow when you start your fasting journey. Below are safety tips to ensure that your experience with intermittent fasting is smooth and seamless.

1. Make Fasting Periods Short

The duration of your fast is solely up to you. There are several techniques to choose from, so just select one that aligns with your lifestyle and daily living. Most regimens you have learned advise 8 to 24 hours of fasting. However, you can fast up to 72 hours if your doctor signals it is safe.

Remember that the longer your fasting window, the higher the risk of the side effects of fasting. Some of these include irritability, dehydration, hunger, fatigue, mood changes, fainting, and inability to focus.

The best thing is to stick to shorter fasting windows to avoid the side effects. This is especially important for you as a beginner and an older person. If you are confident in increasing your fasting time, ensure you seek your primary healthcare consultant's supervision.

• Eat Small Portions on Fast Days

Generally, the idea of fasting is to halt food and drink consumption for a specified period. When you start fasting, don't overcompensate for this by upping your regular food intake. Remember that intermittent fasting plans are based on calorie restriction. Therefore, eat as you usually do during your eating window.

Also, don't go for a full-blown fast where you eat nothing within your fast day. It is much safer to consume small amounts of food during fasting days. Taking this approach helps to lessen the risks associated with fasting. Fasting is also more sustainable since you are less likely to feel hungry.

• Drink Water and Stay Hydrated

Not drinking enough water can lead to dehydration, which can, in turn, lead to thirst, fatigue, and headaches. So, it is crucial to get enough fluid while fasting. Health authorities generally recommend following the 8x8 rule, so you drink 8-0unces glasses of water every day. That is under 2 liters, and it will help you stay hydrated.

But know that the amount of fluid needed by the body can vary according to individuals. Still, most people's needs will likely fall in this range. Because up to 30 percent of required fluid comes from food, you can quickly become dehydrated while fasting.

On a fast, aim to drink two to three liters of water through the course of the day. Still, listen to your body to know when you are thirsty and need to drink more water.

• Try Walking or Meditation

It's challenging to avoid food during fasting windows, mainly if you are bored and hungry. If you don't play your cards right, you might break your fast unintentionally. One surefire way of preventing that is to keep yourself busy with brief walks or meditation.

These activities may help distract you from hunger without using too much of your energy. In general, any activity that is calming and mildly strenuous works because it will keep your mind engaged. You could read a book, listen to a podcast, or take a bath.

• Don't Overeat When You Break Your Fast

Unless you follow the warrior diet, you have no reason to consume a huge meal after the restriction is lifted. Even if you are on the warrior diet, you shouldn't necessarily "feast." Doing that can leave you feeling tired and bloated.

Also, feasting during eating windows can affect your long-term goals by inhibiting or slowing down your progress. As explained in an earlier chapter, your weight is affected by your total calorie quota. Thus, excessive calorie intake after a fast can decrease your calorie deficit.

Stick to your regular healthy eating routine even when you break a fast.

• Stop Fasting if You Don't Feel Great

It is normal to feel tired, irritable, and hunger during fasting windows – but feeling unwell isn't acceptable. If you are new to fasting, limit the restriction to below 24 hours. Keep a snack nearby if you feel faint or unwell.

If you become concerned about your health, stop fasting immediately. You might have to seek medical help if you experience severe tiredness or weakness to where you can't perform your daily tasks. Also, check for feelings of discomfort and sickness.

• Don't Work Out Too Hard

You might be able to maintain your standard exercise program while on a fast. That depends on you. But as a beginner to fasting, you are advised to keep exercise to the lowest intensity you can. Doing this will give insight into how much you can manage.

Low-intensity exercises such as mild yoga, walking, stretching, and housework are ideal for IF beginners. The most vital thing is to listen to your body. Rest if you experience any difficulty with exercise while on a fast. Keep your workout regimen as mild as needed.

Day 1-5 of Fasting

The steps below cover the first five days of fasting and what you should do during this period. This is specifically for the 16:8 plan, but you can tweak it to apply to the methods you want to follow.

Day 1: Don't Eat After Dinner

Eat as naturally as you do throughout the day but stop consuming anything once dinner is over. After dinner at 7 p.m., you are unlikely to be hungry around 8 to 9 p.m. But if you usually lounge around to watch TV or hang out with loved ones after dinner, you might nibble some popcorn, ice cream, or chips.

The tips below will help you through the night:

- Brush your teeth before bed. The minty taste from your toothpaste can help suppress cravings. Brushing also sends a subtle message to your brain you have finished eating, or you'll have to brush again. This creates enough of a barrier to keep you from eating.

- Drink a warm cup of herbal tea or a glass of water if you feel slightly hungry. The effect is calming.

- Go to bed and sleep the hunger off.

Day 2: Delay Breakfast

From the time you slept to the time you wake, you have effectively completed a 12-hour fast – but don't end it just yet. You have only balanced the ratio to 50:50, which is a good thing. That phase is straightforward, so you shouldn't feel it anyway.

It is morning, and there is the usual rush to get out of the house as soon as possible. Unless you work from home, the morning rush is a constant. You don't want to be late, so you grab something to eat on the go or eat as fast as possible. But when fasting, don't do this.

Delay your breakfast so you can eat when it is convenient, instead of rushing it. To make up for the delay, have a couple of glasses of water, coffee, or tea. You might think delaying breakfast is extreme or unhealthy, but it works.

Wait until you have settled in at work or dropped the kids off at school instead of eating amidst the early morning rush. Before you break your fast, check your mail, plan your day, and look at your calendar. Do not sneak in breakfast in the middle of these activities.

Once it is around 10 a.m., you can conveniently have your breakfast without all the chaos. Or, if you feel like you can manage, wait till 11 a.m. before you eat. But if you do eat around 10 a.m., you are unlikely to be hungry during lunchtime. Even though your clock says it's mealtime, your body might not agree. So, wait until you feel hungry again.

Around 2 p.m., you should be hungry; then you can have a nice lunch. Wait until 7 p.m. to have dinner. Then, repeat the steps above: don't eat after dinner and delay your breakfast until 10 a.m.

Day 3: Don't Snack

You have successfully completed a 15-hour fast. Your fasting window started after 7 p.m. the previous night. You ate nothing after dinner, and you delayed gratification (breakfast) until 10 a.m. That equals a whopping 15-hour fast, which is excellent for a beginner. After lunch on the third day, consume nothing until dinnertime. Leave snacks out of it.

• Dinner is just a few hours from lunch, so you can eat very soon. You only need to wait until 7 p.m.

• Hunger is temporary because it comes in waves. That means it will only subside the longer you go without food. It doesn't get worse.

- Sometimes, hunger is an illusion. It isn't real. You are not hungry – it might just be a snacking habit. Or maybe you are just hungry. You might be stressed, anxious, sad, bored, all of which can compel you to eat. Suppress the urge by drinking water, tea, or coffee instead.

- Keep yourself busy. Complete a task, go for a walk, meditate, or call a friend. Before you realize it, it will be time to head home and have your dinner.

Once you get home, cook your meal and eat at 7 p.m. Again, follow the previous steps: skip dinner, delay breakfast until 10 a.m., and don't snack until it's time for dinner.

Day 4: Skip Breakfast

By day 4, you have completed another 15-hour fast without snacking between meals. On the fourth day, skip breakfast by delaying mealtime for one more hour. This means having your first meal of the day at 11 a.m., making it lunch.

Repeat all the tips you have learned so far:

- Practice mindful eating by doing everything you need to do before your meal.

- Wait until you truly feel hungry before eating. Don't eat out of habit, thirst, or emotion.

- Understand that hunger is short-lived. Use tricks to ride hunger waves until they finally go away.

Again, have your dinner at 7 p.m. Repeat the steps you've followed from day 1 of fasting.

Day 5: Repeat

From day 1 to 4, you have built a routine that your body is starting to become familiar with. From day 5, just keep repeating the steps until you complete your plan. The 16:8 method reduces your eating window to one-third of the day, giving you a more generous fasting window to reap the benefits of intermittent fasting.

If you so wish, you can progress to other prolonged variations of intermittent fasting. Regardless of which techniques you choose to follow, always follow the principle of breaking down the fasting time into small, doable steps that can be easily achieved over some time. From there, work your way until you get to the exact point you want.

Fasting is an excellent tool for weight loss, but it can be even greater if you put yourself on a low-carb, high-fat diet while fasting. Its effectiveness depends on how consistent you are in the long run.

Should you follow the steps described in this section, it shouldn't be difficult to achieve consistency. One fun fact about skipping breakfast is that most people aren't starving in the morning, making it easy to skip breakfast without getting extremely hungry.

Chapter Eight: Troubleshooting Intermittent Fasting

Varying factors contribute to how long it may take for you to start losing fat once you start intermittent fasting. Naturally, it varies from person to person, depending on starting weight, intermittent fasting approach taken, types and size of foods consumed during eating windows, and other factors.

Follow everything explained so far in this book by reducing your daily caloric intake and consistently expend more calories than you consume. Weight loss should start from the word "go." However, even though you are shedding the pounds, you may not notice the physical results for a couple of weeks. Most of the time, people just lose "water weight" in the beginner.

Depending on caloric intake during your fasting window, you may lose approximately 1 to 2 pounds each week. Hence, you would have to fast for up to 10 weeks to see any significant change in appearance.

If somehow, you are losing over two pounds per week, that could be a potential red flag. Contact your doctor immediately if you observe that you are losing a considerable amount of weight following a fasting plan. You might need to evaluate your daily or weekly caloric intake to establish that you are consuming enough nutrition to cater to your body's needs.

However, if you don't seem to be losing weight despite sticking to all the fasting guidelines, there could be different reasons. You could be making inevitable mistakes without realizing it. So, what could the mistakes be? Discover below.

High Caloric Intake During Eating Windows

The first likely reason could be that you are consuming too many calories during your eating window. As mentioned several times, weight loss via intermittent fasting boils down to the number of calories that go in versus the ones that come out. If you keep your caloric intake at the same number as before you started fasting, you can't possibly lose weight.

The whole point of intermittent fasting is restricting the time you eat to cut down on your calorie intake. Therefore, you can't keep packing in the same number of calories as before. If you do that, it means you haven't made any changes to your diet.

Solution: To fix this problem, get a calorie-counting app to track your intake for the first few days of intermittent fasting. With an app like that, you will know the exact number of calories you need to consume daily to lose weight. Usually, the estimations aren't wholly accurate, but they can make a difference initially. Some of these apps also have features that let you know the number of calories in most food. That way, you can plan your meal and adjust your diet.

Low Caloric Intake on Non-Fasting Days

Not consuming the required number of calories on non-fasting days makes your body conserve the consumed energy instead of burning it. Therefore, always endeavor to meet the daily caloric requirement on non-fasting days.

Solution: Fix this problem by making a meal plan specifically for your non-fasting days. Make sure the program balances each meal to contain 300 to 500 calories. This way, don't rely on guesswork to determine if you meet the requirements or not. Also, you won't have to skimp on calories for yourself.

Wrong Eating Window

There are different approaches to take toward intermittent fasting. You cannot try all these methods, so you have to choose one consistent with your lifestyle and weight loss goals. If you choose one that does not suit your lifestyle, you might see no fasting results.

For instance, if you typically hit the gym during weekdays or work overtime, the 5:2 diet may be too restrictive for you. At the end of each fasting window, you may end up feeling famished. This is a sure recipe for failure.

Solution: Choose an eating window that falls within the time you do the most strenuous activities in your life. If a 12-hour window is all you can do without triggering significant discomfort feelings, go ahead with it. Don't force yourself to do more than you can handle. You may also start with a 16-hour fast. The steps in the preceding chapter breaks down 16:8 fasting into small steps that make things easy for beginners.

Wrong Food Intake

Just because IF focuses on your mealtime instead of tracking macronutrients does not give you the room to fill your diet up with junk. You must still eat healthy while you are fasting. Eating the wrong food can obstruct your weight loss.

The wrong foods don't give you the nutrients your body needs to sustain itself. Nourishing your body with nutrient-rich whole foods is a must. The body finds those easier to break down during a fasting window, which improves satiation.

Do not use IF as an excuse to consume processed foods and sugar because they are not suitable for your body when it is in a fasted state.

Solution: Fill up your diet with healthy fats, complex carbs, lean protein, and more fiber. Refer back to chapters where the kind of healthy foods to eat during intermittent fasting has been explained. On the side, you can still consume some of your favorite less-healthy foods like ice cream and pizza, but make sure you do this in moderation.

Short Fasting Window

You are unlikely to get any results from an intermittent fasting plan if your fasting window is less than 12 hours a day. Shortening your daily eating window by 1 to 2 hours will make no difference. A short fasting window makes your body unable to complete all the phases in the fed-fast cycle. You need to change much of your regular eating routine.

Solution: To achieve success, you need to have at least a 12-hour fasting window. Most experts recommend a 14-hour window for women because it can be successful for most intermittent dieters. This does not mean you can't start with a longer eating window, but make sure it doesn't outweigh the fasting window. If anything, starting with a longer eating window means you can eventually work your way down as you get more familiar with intermittent fasting.

Meal-Skipping During Eating Window

You cannot skip meals during your eating window because that will cause extreme hunger during the fasting periods. That makes you more likely to break your fast. It is best to avoid this. Do not restrict yourself too much during any eating window. Otherwise, you may end up binge-eating the next fasting window. The result of this is too much caloric intake.

Solution: Eat until you are full during your eating windows, but don't overstuff yourself. Just make sure that you are satisfied. Also consider doing meal preps for the weekdays on weekends. By doing that, you are unlikely to skip meals even when you get busy or throw off your daily schedule.

Intense Workout

Often, many people mistake starting their intermittent fasting plan around the same time they just jump onto a new exercise regimen. Some boost their current plan because they believe that will help increase the rate at which they lose fat. Things do not work like that.

An intense workout while you are reducing your food intake is not ideal. Over-exercising while fasting causes your energy levels to drop as your hunger levels rapidly increase. You may consume more calories than you can expend during your eating window. Even with the intense exercise plan, don't be surprised if you get no noticeable changes.

Solution: Keep exercise light during fasting periods. If you are on the 5:2 plan, don't exercise during your fasting days. In general, make sure that you follow a challenging workout program, but make it enjoyable. If you feel ravenous on the days you exercise, it may mean you are overworking.

Insufficient Hydration

The importance of drinking enough water on fasting days cannot be overstated. Not getting enough fluid intake while you are on a fast can leave you feeling dehydrated. By not drinking sufficient water, you also miss out on the amazing benefits of water regarding satiating or suppressing hunger.

Solution: Drink 2 to 3 liters of water daily during fasting and non-fasting windows. And the best thing is that you can add some flavor to your fluid intake. Hot tea, iced tea, black coffee tea, stevia coffee, and seltzer water are some drinks that are approved for intermittent fasting. These drinks are non-caloric, meaning they won't add to your calorie intake no matter how much you drink them in a day.

Deviating From the Plan

Following an IF plan may be difficult for beginners who are not familiar with prolonged periods without eating anything. If you keep cheating on your plan or cutting corners because of hunger, it won't yield your expected results. It is much better to reevaluate yourself and your lifestyle to determine if time-restricted eating is for you or not.

Solution: Choose an IF plan that matches your lifestyle perfectly. That increases the likelihood of you following the plan consistently - despite obstacles.

Those are the most common problems people face when they start intermittent fasting. Suppose you address these problems and apply the solutions offered for each. In that case, you will start seeing noticeable changes in your body with your intermittent fasting plan.

As you continue fasting, you will learn some lessons that will change your perception about intermittent fasting and help build you into a better dieter and faster. What are these lessons?

The first lesson you might learn is that mindset is single-handedly your biggest obstacle. This dieting plan is simple and straightforward. Many people agree that it is one of the most straightforward dieting strategies to follow. All you have to do is *not eat until you wake up, eat once you get to work, eat again during lunch hours, and go about your business until dinner arrives again.*

But there is a mental barrier most people face when they attempt fasting. "Will it affect my thinking if I don't eat?" "If I don't eat, will I faint or fall sick?" "What will it be like? Can I do this?" These are some thoughts that run to and from your mind when you get started.

If you get past this mental barrier and questions, you will realize that nothing happens. Life will continue as before. You may not even feel like someone who has just made a huge lifestyle change. The only apparent difference will be the extra pounds falling off your body each week as your fasting progresses.

The things you have convinced yourself about, such as the hours you should eat or snack are perceptions. They don't matter in context. You eat breakfast at 7 a.m. because you were told to, not because you actually have to.

Forget what you think you know and readjust your mental space to accommodate your new lifestyle. The ability to think and act differently is the foundation to success in anything you try.

A second lesson you should expect to learn is that weight loss is easy. That is right – because eating less frequently means eating less overall. Because of this, most people on this diet end up losing fat.

Intermittent fasting offers you a simple way of cutting down on your weight by cutting down on total caloric intake without making a drastic change to your diet. And this is why many dieters enjoy fasting.

Even if you follow a plan that lets you eat two large meals at lunch and dinner, you end up consuming fewer calories than you usually would if you had three regular meals with snacks between.

Yes, muscle loss happens as you get older, but you might just be surprised at the results you see when you start time-restricted eating. If you follow your plan as you should, you may build and maintain your muscle mass which means you are burning fat rather than muscle.

There are several other personal lessons you will learn as you progress with your journey. Incorporate these into your life as you work on making intermittent fasting an integral part of your daily routine. Remember that intermittent fasting is more than just a dieting technique – it is a lifestyle.

Chapter Nine: Exercises for Women Over 50

Chapter 5 mentioned that strength training, stability training, aerobic training, and flexibility training are a must in a workout routine for women over 50. While intermittent fasting helps you lose weight, you can improve your body with exercise the older you get. In other words, the right exercise regimen can help you turn back the years on your whole appearance.

Several studies have shown that exercise slows down the physiological aging clock and helps older people stay young. And although cardiovascular activities like walking, biking, cycling, and jogging are great for your heart and lung health, strength training is the real deal that provides what your body needs in its fifties.

Strength training is the best exercise for you because it helps you stay younger and more vital and keeps you functioning optimally as your body ages. To remain vibrant and self-sufficient for many more years to come, the strength training exercise below is your key to achieving that.

Experts recommend strength-training for older women because, after 50, the crucial things shift from building big biceps or achieving flat abs to maintaining a strong, lean, and healthy body that is less susceptible to injury and diseases.

Strength-training workouts can help you build bone density, add muscle mass, shed body fat, and improve your cognitive health. They also reduce the risk of chronic illnesses. These reasons explain why strength-training is a big deal for older women.

Even if you do only 20 to 30 minutes of training per day, you can notice considerable changes in your overall appearance and mental health. It often helps to have a physically active group of friends to exercise with. Check out workout classes in your local area, or simply bring friends together.

If you can afford to talk to a fitness expert, then speak to one – even if it is just for a session. In a single session, they can teach the proper form and how to move your body appropriately when trying strength-training workouts.

Forearm Plank

This exercise targets your shoulders and abdominals.

1. Start by lying on the floor. Let your forearms spread flat while your elbows are placed directly under your shoulders.

2. Raise your body off the ground and engage your core as you do this. Ensure that your forearms stay on the floor and your entire body forms a straight line from head to feet. Keep your core engaged, and don't let your hips move out of position. They should neither dip nor rise.

3. Hold still for 3o seconds instead of doing reps. If you feel uncomfortable or your lower back hurts, places your knees on the ground.

Modified Push-Up

This workout targets your shoulders, core, and arms.

1. Start in a kneeling position on a workout mat. Place both hands below your shoulders with your knees behind your hips. That way, your back takes an angled and long-form.

2. Tuck your toes under, tighten your core and slightly bend your elbows. Then slowly lower your chest toward the ground.

3. Look straight at the front of your fingertips, so the neck stays long.

4. Press your chest back to the initial position. Repeat these steps a few times.

Stability Ball Chest Fly

This workout targets your chest, back, glutes, and abdominals.

1. Hold two dumbbells to your chest. Position your shoulder blades and head directly on top of the stability ball. Keep the rest of your body in a tabletop pose. Check to see that your feet are hip-distance apart.

2. Raise the pair of dumbbells together straight above your chest, with the palms facing each other.

3. Slowly lower your arms out to the sides while slightly bending your elbows until they are about chest level.

4. Tighten your chest and bring your hands together back to the top.

Basic Squat

The basic squat workout is targeted at the glutes, hamstrings, and quads.

1. Stand upright with your feet apart. Maintain a hip-distance between both while your hips, knees, and toes all face forward. Hold a pair of dumbbells in both hands to increase the difficulty.

2. Stretch your buttocks outward as you bend your knees. Do this as if you are trying to sit on a chair. Ensure your knees are behind your toes and shift the weight on your heels.

3. Rise back up and repeat the workout a couple of times.

Shoulder Overhead Press

This workout is targeted at your biceps, back, and shoulders.

1. Pull your feet hip-distance apart. Bring your elbows out to your sides as you create a goal post position. Keep your dumbbells at the side of your head and tighten your abdominal muscles.

2. Slowly press the dumbbells until your arms are up straight. Return to the initial position with slow control. You can try this workout on a chair or a stability ball with your feet wide apart.

These five strength-training exercises are some of the easiest to perform. Incorporate one or two into your day-to-day workout routine.

Aerobic training makes a lot of difference to your workout programs. They exercise the large muscles in your body, which benefits your cardiovascular system and weight. Get in 20 minutes of aerobic exercise each training session, at least three days a week. Ensure that you pass the "talk test" when training. The "talk test" means working out at a pace that simultaneously allows you to have a conversation.

Stretching exercises are equally as important as strength training and aerobic training. It is a good idea to stretch a few times every day. The American College of Sports Medicine recommends stretching your major muscle groups two to three times a week at 60 seconds per exercise.

The point of stretches is to help you stay flexible as you get older. This improves mobility. Daily stretches can help your hips and hamstrings remain flexible despite aging. If your posture is causing any form of problem, form a habit of stretching your muscle groups every day. Also, if you sit at a desk all day, stretching can help lower back pain.

Simple Back Stretch

This simple stretching exercise is also called the "Standing cat camel." It is an excellent work-related stretch that can be completed in four easy steps.

1. Stand with your feet apart and your knees slightly bent. Make sure the distance between your feet is shoulder-width

2. Lean slightly forward with your hands just above your knees

3. Round your back to close your chest and curve your shoulders forward

4. Arch your back to open your chest and roll your shoulders backward

5. Repeat steps 1-4 multiple times

If you work a job that keeps you in the same position most of the time, consider trying the 2 minutes breaks to reverse the posture every 60 to 120 minutes.

Static Cat-Camel

A static stretch is when you stretch a muscle group to the fullest and hold it for about 15 to 30 seconds instead of repetitions. There is no harm in doing static stretches as long as you don't overdo them by remaining static until your muscles start to hurt. Below is a static version of the standing cat camel.

1. Lace your fingers together and turn your palms outwards in front of you

2. Curve your back and shoulders forward and reach your arms as far as you can with your palms

3. Hold still for 10 to 20 seconds

4. Now, release your fingers from one another, and twist your wrists behind your back gently

5. Raise your arms as high as they can behind your back. Do that without freeing your wrists so your shoulders roll back as your chest opens

Whether you are trying the static or dynamic stretch, you should never feel pain. What you should feel at any point is a stretch. So, don't stretch yourself beyond the range of motion your body needs.

Besides the strength-training and flexibility training exercises, you can try other workouts like the ones below.

Aerobic Interval Training

Aerobic interval training involves alternating between modern-to-high-intensity workouts with a recovery interval and a work interval. Your work interval is typically below 85 percent of the maximum heart rate. The recovery interval should bring your heart rate down to 110 bpm as you rest.

You can try this interval training with any aerobic activity of your choice, such as walking, running, jogging, or cycling. You can do it for 10 to 60 minutes. If you are new to interval training, do it for 10 minutes with a 2-minute recovery period.

Below is an AIT workout to try:

1. Warm-up your body for up to 10 minutes comfortably

2. Pick up speed or exertion to recovery level for 3 minutes

3. Increase speed for 1 to 2 minutes to increase your heart rate, but be careful not to exceed the 85% maximum heart rate

4. Return to recovery speed for 2 to 5 minutes

5. Repeat the work and recovery intervals during your chosen training length

You can try AITs two or more times each week.

Bicycle Crunch

The bicycle crunch is a classic exercise that works all of your core muscles at once, particularly the obliques and rectus abdominus. Try this exercise by following the steps below.

1. Lay flat on the floor and press your lower back to the ground

2. Place your hands behind your head gently without yanking your neck

3. Raise one of your knees to a 45-degree angle and let the other remain straight

4. Shift your legs back and forth as you would if you were cycling. Alternatively, extend one knee as you lift the other.

5. Touch your left elbow to your right knee and right elbow to left knee each time

6. Complete at least 20 to 50 reps on both sides. Be deliberate with your movements and remain steady.

7. Rest and complete two more sets before you wrap up

As you get stronger, up the number of reps you complete per set.

The Bridge

The bridge exercise targets your lower back, hamstrings, and gluteus muscles (buttocks). It can help improve spine stability and abdominal strength.

1. To assume the position, lie flat on your back and bend your knees. Keep your feet balanced and position your arms by your sides.

2. Inhale slowly and tighten your core and glutes while you lift your hips to form a straight line between your knees and shoulders.

3. Remain in the position for 15 to 60 seconds without dropping your lower back or buttocks.

4. If you feel like increasing this exercise's intensity, lift your leg as high as possible and hold still for 10 seconds.

As you become better at this exercise with practice, start increasing the duration of the pose.

Every bit of movement counts when you are in your 50s. If you find yourself too busy to commit to a standard workout program, find other ways to increase motion. All the extra steps you take add up to significant weight loss and overall health benefits.

Here are some ideas you can adopt to be in motion always:

• Take a dog for daily walks.

• Abandon the elevator and start using the stairs. Don't shout at people from the stairs – seize that opportunity to go on up.

• Get up whenever you have to talk with co-workers. Don't send texts or emails. Try walking to meetings regularly.

- Make brisk walking a habit – do it whenever you can. Always take comfortable shoes with you. That way, your feet can serve as your primary mode of transit.

Find a game, sport, or activity that requires mild to intense physical activity levels and make it your newest hobby. It is easy to commit to workout regimens when doing things you consider enjoyable.

Chapter Ten: Recipes for Intermittent Fasting

Whether your eating window is within a 12-hour, 8-hour, or 4-hour range, you need to consume whole foods with powerful nutrients that can keep you feeling full and satisfied throughout your fasting window. The best approach is to try low-carb-high-protein recipes sure to make you feel nourished.

Naturally, you have to try different recipes for breakfast, lunch, and dinner. So, one by one, here are recipes ideal for different phases of your eating window.

Egg Scramble and Sweet Potatoes

Total cooking time: 25 minutes

Servings: 1

Ingredients:

- 1 sweet potato, diced
- Half cup of chopped onions
- Salt
- Pepper

- 2 tsp chopped rosemary

- 4 big eggs

- 2 spoons chopped chive

Directions:

1. Preheat your oven to 425 degrees Fahrenheit. Toss the diced potato, chopped onion, rosemary, salt, and pepper on a baking sheet. Apply cooking spray and allow to roast until soft and tender, for about 20 minutes.

2. Meanwhile, whisk the eggs and egg whites in a medium-sized bowl. Add a pinch of salt and pepper. Spritz with cooking oil and scramble the eggs in 5 minutes.

3. Sprinkle chopped chives and eat with the spuds.

One serving has 580 calories, 52g carbs, 44g protein, 9g fiber, and 20g fat.

PB & J Overnight Oats

Total time: 5 minutes (plus 8 hours for refrigeration)

Servings: 1

Ingredients:

- ¼ cup of fast-cooking rolled oats

- ½ cup of 2% milk

- ¼ cup of mashed raspberries

- 3 tablespoons of creamy peanut butter

Directions:

1. Add the oats, milk, mashed raspberries, and peanut butter together in a fairly-sized bowl. Stir gently until silky smooth.

2. Cover and put inside the refrigerator overnight. The next day, uncover and use whole raspberries as toppings.

One serving contains 455 calories, 36g carbs, 20g protein, 9g fiber, and 28g fat.

Turkish Egg Breakfast

Total time: 13 minutes

Servings: 2

Ingredients:

- 2 tablespoons olive oil
- ¾ cup of red bell pepper, diced
- ¾ cup eggplant, diced
- Pinch of salt and pepper
- 5 large eggs
- ¼ teaspoon paprika
- 1 whole-wheat pita
- 2 dollops plain yogurt
- Chopped cilantro

Directions:

1. Put a large nonstick skillet on moderate-high heat. Heat the olive oil. Add in the eggplant, bell pepper, salt, and pepper. Sauté until tender for about 7 minutes.

2. Lightly beat the eggs. Then, stir in the eggs and paprika. Add a little more salt and pepper to taste. Allow to cook and regularly stir until the eggs are scrambled.

3. Sprinkle the chopped cilantro and serve with one dollop of yogurt and pita.

One serving contains 470 calories, 26g carbs, 25g protein, 4g fiber, and 29g fat.

Almond Apple Spice Muffins

Total time: 15 minutes

Servings: 5

Ingredients:

- ½ stick butter

- 4 scoops of vanilla protein powder

- 2 cups of almond meal

- 4 eggs

- 1 cup of unsweetened applesauce

- 1 teaspoon allspice

- 1 tablespoon cinnamon

- 1 teaspoon cloves

- 2 tablespoons baking powder

Directions:

1. Preheat oven to 350 degrees. Using a small microwave-fitting bowl, melt the stick butter on low heat for about 30 seconds.

2. Thoroughly mix the remaining ingredients with the melted butter in a relatively large bowl—spritz two muffin tins with the cooking spray. If you have cupcake liners, use those.

3. Pour the mixture into muffin tins without overfilling. You should get ten muffins.

4. Put a tray in the oven and bake for 10 to 12 minutes. Do not overbake as this can make the muffins go too dry. Once baked, eject the tray from the oven. Put in the second tray and let the rest of the muffins bake the same way.

One serving contains 485 calories, 16g carbs, 40g protein: 5 g fiber, and 31g fat.

Greek Chickpea Waffles

Total time: 30 minutes

Servings: 2

Ingredients:

- ¾ cup of chickpea flour

- ½ teaspoon salt

- ½ teaspoon baking soda

- ¾ cup plain Greek yogurt (2%)

- 6 eggs

- Salt and pepper

- Tomatoes, olive oil, cucumbers, parsley, scallion, yogurt, lemon juice for serving (optional)

Directions:

1. Preheat oven to 200 degrees. Get a rimmed baking sheet and place a wire rack over to – put in the oven, heat one waffle irons per directions.

2. Beat together the flour, soda, and salt in a large bowl. In a different small bowl, beat together the egg and Greek yogurt. Mix the wet ingredients into the dry ones.

3. Softly cover the iron waffle with cooking spray, preferably a nonstick one. In groups, drop ¼ cup batter into each iron waffle section and cook until it turns to a golden-brown color. This will take around 4 to 5 minutes. Move the waffles to the oven to warm. Repeat with the rest of the batter.

4. Serve your waffles with a delicious tomato dressing or a simple mix of nut butter and berries.

One serving contains 415 calories, 24g carbs, 35g protein, 4g fiber, and 18g fat.

Turmeric Tofu Scramble

Total time: 15 minutes

Servings: 1

Ingredients:

- 1 portobello mushroom
- 3 cherry tomatoes
- 1 tablespoon olive oil
- 14-oz firm tofu
- Salt and pepper
- ¼ teaspoon ground turmeric
- A pinch of garlic powder
- ½ avocado, sliced thinly

Directions:

1. Preheat oven to 400 degrees. Place the mushroom and tomatoes on a baking sheet. Brush with olive oil. Add salt and pepper to season. Allow to roast until soft and tender – 10 minutes should do.

2. Additionally, add the tofu, garlic powder, turmeric, and a pinch of salt together in a moderately-sized bowl. Mash together with a fork.

3. Add 1 tablespoon olive oil to a large skillet. Pour in the mashed tofu mixture and let it cook. Stir until it takes a firm and egg-like form. This should be around 3 minutes.

4. Dish the tofu and serve with the roasted mushroom, tomatoes, and, if you like, avocado.

One serving contains 430 calories, 17g carbs, 21g protein, 8g fiber, and 33g fat.

Avocado Ricotta Power Toast

Total time: 5 minutes

Servings: 1

Ingredients:

- 1 whole-grain bread, sliced
- ¼ smashed avocado
- Pinch of crushed red pepper flakes
- 2 tablespoon ricotta
- Pinch flaky sea salt

Directions:

1. Toast the bread

2. Add avocado, crushed pepper flakes, ricotta, and sea salt as toppings

3. Serve with scrambled eggs, with a serving of fruit or yogurt

One serving contains 290 calories, 29g carbs, 10g protein, 10g fiber, and 17fg fat.

Apple and Cheddar Plus Mixed Greens

Total time: 5 minutes

Servings: 1

Ingredients:

- 2 tablespoon olive oil
- ¾ cup balsamic vinegar
- ¾ teaspoon ground black pepper
- ¼ teaspoon onion powder
- ¾ teaspoon garlic powder

- A pinch of salt

- 1 cup apple and cheddar

- 1 medium banana

- 2 cups mixed greens

- 1 tablespoon peanut butter

Directions

1. Mix the first five ingredients together in a medium-sized jar. Close the jar and shake it vibrantly until all the ingredients have mixed together well. Put in the refrigerator until it is lunchtime.

2. Chop the apple and cheddar cheese into cubes. Add the mixed greens together in a mixing bowl. Toss to mix together

3. Serve salad with a drizzle of vinaigrette

One serving contains 630 calories, 50g carbs, 10g protein, 6g fiber, and 47g fat.

Turkey Tacos

Total time: 25 minutes

Servings: 4

Ingredients:

- 2 teaspoons oil

- 1 finely chopped clove garlic

- 1 chopped red onion, small

- 1 tablespoon sodium-free taco seasoning

- 1 lb. lean turkey, ground

- 8 warmed whole-grain corn tortillas

- 1 sliced avocado

- ¼ cup of sour cream

- ½ cup Mexican cheese, shredded

- 1 cup lettuce, chopped

- Salsa, for serving

Directions:

1. Put a large skillet on medium-high to heat the oil. Pour in the onion and stir for 5 minutes until tender. Add the garlic and let it cook for 1 minute.

2. Pour in the turkey and allow to cook. Break up with a spoon at intervals until it is nearly brown, for about 5 minutes. Add a cup of water, plus the taco seasoning. Allow simmering until the water is reduced by more than half. This should take 7 minutes.

3. Fill up the corn tortillas with the turkey and use the sour cream, salsa, avocado, lettuce, and cheese as toppings.

One serving contains 470 calories, 30g carbs, 28g protein, 6g fiber, and 27g fat.

Chicken with Fried Cauliflower Rice

Total time: 35 minutes

Servings: 4

Ingredients:

- 2 tablespoon grapeseed oil

- 1 lb. pounded boneless, skinless chicken breast

- Eggs, beaten

- 2 finely chopped red bell peppers

- 1 finely chopped onion

- 2 carrots, finely chopped

- 2 finely chopped cloves of garlic

- 4 finely-chopped scallions, plus more for serving

- 4 cups of cauliflower rice

- ½ cup of thawed frozen peas

- 2 teaspoons of soy sauce, low sodium

- 2 teaspoons of rice vinegar

- Kosher salt and pepper, for taste

Directions:

1. Use a large, deep skillet that is over moderate-high. Heat the oil. Add the chicken breast and cook until it turns golden brown. This should take 3 or 4 minutes for both sides. Move chicken to a cutting board and allow to cool for 6 minutes before slicing. Add 1 tablespoon oil to the skillet. Pour in the eggs and aim for scrambled until you get the right set. Move to a bowl.

2. In the skillet, add the carrot, onion, and bell pepper and cook. Stir frequently until softened. Mix in the garlic and let it cook for 1 minute. Toss in the peas and scallions.

3. Add soy sauce, cauliflower, rice vinegar, salt, and pepper. Toss gently to mix all together. Allow the cauliflower "rice" to sit until it starts to brown. Do not stir.

4. Toss in the sliced chicken and scrambled eggs.

One serving contains 430 calories, 25g carbs, 45g protein, 7g fiber, and 16g fat.

Healthy Spaghetti Bolognese

Total time: 60 minutes

Servings: 4

Ingredients:

- 1 spaghetti squash, large
- ½ teaspoon garlic powder
- 2 tablespoon olive oil
- 1 finely chopped onion, small
- Kosher salt and pepper
- 1 ¼ lb. ground turkey
- 4 finely chopped cloves of garlic
- 3 cups of fresh tomato, diced
- 8 ounces of sliced cremini mushrooms
- 8 ounces of low-sodium, sugar-free tomato sauce
- Fresh basil, chopped

Directions:

1. Heat the oven to 400 degrees. Split the spaghetti squash in half and discard the seeds. Rub both halves with ½ teaspoon of oil each and add garlic powder and salt and pepper (1/4 tsp) to season. Put the skin side on a baking sheet (rimmed) and allows to cook until softened. This should take up to 4o minutes. After cooking, allow cooking for 10 minutes.

2. In the meantime, put a large skillet on moderate-high, and heat the remaining oil. Add the chopped onions and season with ¼ teaspoons of salt and pepper (each) and cook until softened for 6 minutes. Stir as it cooks.

3. Add turkey to the mix and break it up into smaller pieces as it cooks. Do this for about 7 minutes until browned. Put in the garlic, stir, and let it cook for 1 minute.

4. Gently push the mixture to one side and pour in the mushrooms on another side. Cook for 5 minutes until tender. Stir as it cooks. Mix together with the turkey. Pour in the tomatoes and tomato sauce. Leave it to simmer for 8 to 10 minutes.

5. Meanwhile, scoop out the spaghetti squash and serve on a plate. Scoop the turkey Bolognese over it and sprinkle the chopped basil if you wish.

One serving contains 45 calories, 31g carb, 32g protein, 6g fiber, and 23g fat.

Sheet Pan Steak

Total time: 50 minutes

Servings: 4

Ingredients:

- 1 lb. cremini mushrooms (small), trimmed and split into halves
- 1 ¼ lb. bunch broccolini, halved and trimmed
- 4 finely chopped cloves of garlic
- ¼ teaspoon of red pepper flakes
- 3 tablespoons of olive oil
- Kosher salt and pepper
- 1 ½ lb. New York strip steaks, trimmed
- 1 can low-sodium cannellini beans

Directions:

1. Preheat oven to 450 degrees. Using a large, rimmed baking sheet, toss the broccolini, mushrooms, oil, garlic, red pepper flakes, and salt and pepper. Put the sheet into the oven and allow to roast tenderly for 15 minutes.

2. Push the sheet containing the mushroom mixture to the edge to allow enough room for the steaks.

3. Add ¼ teaspoon of salt and pepper to the steaks to the season—place at the center of the pan. Roast the steaks until done to satisfaction. For medium-rare, roast for 7 minutes. Move the steaks to your cutting board and cool off for 5 minutes before you slice.

4. Rinse the beans and move them to the baking sheet. Toss to mix together. Allow roasting until thoroughly heated.

5. Serve the beans and vegetables with sliced steaks.

One serving is 465 calories, 26g carbs, 42g protein, 8g fiber, and 22g fat.

Wild Cajun Spiced Salmon

Total: 30 minutes

Servings: 4

Ingredients:

- 1 lb. Salmon Fillet, wild Alaskan
- ½ cauliflower head, cut into florets
- 1 broccoli head, cut into florets
- 3 tablespoons olive oil
- ½ teaspoon of garlic powder
- 4 tomatoes, medium and diced
- Sodium-free taco seasoning

Directions:

1. Preheat oven to 375 degrees. Put the salmon fillet in a reasonably large baking dish. Mix the taco seasoning with ½ cup of water in a smaller bowl. Add the mixture over the salmon and let it bake until thoroughly opaque. Do this for 12 to 15 minutes.

2. Meanwhile, use a food processor to pulse the broccoli and cauliflower until thoroughly chopped and "riced."

3. Put a large skillet on medium-high. Pour in the oil to heat. Put in the broccoli and cauliflower, then sprinkle the garlic powder. Toss and cook until softened. That should take 6 minutes.

4. Serve the salmon on the rice and add the tomatoes as toppings.

One serving contains 410 calories, 9g carbs, 42g protein, 3g fiber, and 23g fat.

Pork Chops with Bloody Mary Tomato Salad

Total time: 25 minutes

Servings: 4

Ingredients

- 2 tablespoons red wine vinegar
- 2 tablespoons olive oil
- 2 teaspoons dry-squeezed horseradish
- 2 teaspoons of Worcestershire sauce
- ½ teaspoon tabasco
- Kosher salt
- ½ teaspoon of celery seeds
- 1 pint of halved cherry tomatoes

- 2 thinly-sliced celery stalks

- ½ finely-sliced red onion, small

- Pepper

- 4 (2 ¼ lb.) small pork chops

- 1 little green-leaf lettuces, with torn leaves

- ¼ cup finely-chopped flat-leaf parsley

Directions:

1. Heat your grill to moderate-high. Using a large bowl, mix the oil, vinegar, horseradish, Worcestershire sauce, Tabasco, celery seeds, salt together. Toss the tomatoes, onion, and celery together.

2. Add ½ teaspoon salt and pepper to the pork chops to season. Grill for 5 to 7 minutes on each side until cooked and golden brown.

3. Fold the parsley inside the tomatoes and dish over the pork and greens.

4. Serve with potatoes or mashed cauliflower.

One serving contains 400 calories, 8g carbs, 39g protein, 3g fiber, and 23g fat.

Pork Tenderloin with Butternut Squash and Brussels Sprouts

Total time: 50 minutes

Servings: 4

Ingredients:

- 1 ¾ trimmed pork tenderloin

- Pepper

- Salt

- 2 sprigs thyme, fresh

- 3 tablespoon canola oil

- 2 peeled garlic cloves

- 4 cups butternut squash, diced

- 4 cups of halved and cut Brussels sprouts

Directions:

1. Preheat oven to 4oo degrees. Put the tenderloin in a large bowl and season all over with salt and pepper. Put a big iron cast pan on medium-high heat and pour in 1 tablespoon oil. Heat until it shimmers, then add in the tenderloin and stir until it turns golden brown on every side. This should take up to 12 minutes—dish into a plate.

2. Add the garlic, thyme, and remaining oil to the pan and cook until the aroma comes out for 1 minute. Pour in the Brussels sprouts, butternut squash, and a large pinch of salt and pepper. Cook and occasionally stir for about 6 minutes until the veggies are slightly browned.

3. Put the tenderloin over the vegetables and place everything inside the oven. Allow roasting until the veggies are tender and the tenderloin is thoroughly cooked. You could insert a meat thermometer into the tenderloin to check the degree. It should be up to 140 degrees.

4. Put on oven mittens and take out the pan from the oven. Let the tenderloin cool off for 5 minutes before you slice and serve with the tender vegetables. Toss the greens with balsamic vinegar to serve as a side dish.

One serving contains 400 calories, 25g carbs, 44g protein, 6g fiber, and 15g fat.

Grilled Lemon Salmon

Total time: 27 minutes

Servings: 4

Ingredients:

- ½ teaspoon pepper
- 2 teaspoons fresh dill
- ½ teaspoon garlic powder
- ½ teaspoon salt
- ½ lbs. salmon fillets
- 1 chicken bouillon cube
- ¼ cup of brown sugar
- 3 tablespoons water
- 3 tablespoons oil
- 3 tablespoons soy sauce
- 4 finely chopped green onions
- 1 thinly-sliced lemon
- 2 ring-sliced onions

Directions:

1. Sprinkle the fresh dill, salt, pepper, and garlic powder over the salmon fillet.

2. Put inside a shallow glass pan

3. Add the chicken bouillon, soy sauce, sugar, and green onions together. Mix thoroughly.

4. Pour the mixture over the salmon fillet

5. Cover for 1 hour and allow to chill.

6. Drain the marinade

7. Place on preheated grill on medium heat with the lemon and oil over it.

8. Cover and allow to cook for 15 minutes or until the fish is done.

One serving contains 285 calories, 7.1 carbs, 20.3g protein, 0.5g fiber, and 19.8g fat.

Strawberry-Avocado Smoothie

Servings: 1

- 1 pound of strawberries, fresh or frozen
- 1 ½ cup of unsweetened almond milk
- 1 big, ripe avocado

Blend all the ingredients together until you achieve a smooth and refined taste.

One serving contains 190 calories, 28g carbs, 3g protein, 6g fiber, and 9g fat.

Creamy Chocolate Smoothie with MCT Oil

Servings: 1

- ½ cup of coconut full-fat coconut milk. You may substitute it with heavy whipping cream.
- ½ cup of peeled and seeded avocado
- ½ teaspoon of vanilla extract
- 2 tablespoons of cocoa powder
- Pinch of salt
- ½ cup of ice
- 1 tablespoon of MCT oil (or coconut oil)
- Non-caloric sweetener to taste

Blend all together, minus the ice, until smooth. If needed, add 2 tablespoons of water until you get the desired consistency. Add ice and blend until it becomes creamy.

One serving contains 595 calories, 19g carbs, 10g protein, 11g fiber, and 55g fat.

LCHF Green Protein Smoothie

Servings: 2

- 1 cup of fresh spinach leaves
- 1 ½ teaspoon of freshly-squeezed lemon juice
- ½ cup of peeled and seeded avocado
- 1 tablespoon of MCT oil
- 1 scoop of protein powder, low-carb
- 1 ½ teaspoon of flaxseed powder
- 1 teaspoon vanilla extract
- ¼ cup of water – adjustable as needed
- 5 ice cubes

Mix all the ingredients in the smoothie blender and blend until you get a smooth taste. If you don't consume dairy, please replace the unsweetened almond milk with whatever you want.

One serving contains 140 calories, 8.6g carbs, 4g protein, 3.8g fiber, and 10.8g fat.

Cinnamon Smoothie with Protein

Servings: 1

- 1 cup of unsweetened coconut or almond milk
- 1 scoop of protein powder, low-carb
- 1 tablespoon of MCT oil
- 4 ice cubes
- ½ teaspoon of cinnamon

Mix all ingredients together and blend till it is smooth. For a thicker and creamier consistency, replace ¼ cup of almond milk with ¼ heavy whipped cream.

Incorporate these tasty recipes into your intermittent fasting meal plan to ensure you don't consume too much or too few calories.

One serving contains 160 calories, 31g carbs, 5g protein, 4g fiber, and 3g fat.

Chapter Eleven: Balancing Intermittent Fasting and Your Social Life

Intermittent fasting can have a significant impact on your social life. You may not realize that a considerable aspect of your social life is built on meals and drinks. When you hang out with friends, you have a drink or two. When you have a meeting with coworkers at a restaurant, you eat to your heart's content.

Most of the social activities you engage in with the people in your life revolve around caloric intake. Naturally, this poses a challenge to your intermittent fasting journey. How do you navigate the intricacies of social life without affecting your resolution to meet your weight loss goals with extended fasting?

To maintain a balance between your social life and your weight loss journey, you have to follow only three rules. These rules are simple:

- Compromise
- Undertake
- Explain

The first is "compromise," which you may consider the act of making sacrifices to satisfy another person. It is an integral part of integrating IF perfectly into your social life. As crucial as compromise is, though, it should always come last. Do not resort to it until you have no other choice.

You cannot compromise your fasting every time you have a hangout with friends or family. Doing that all of the time is merely undermining the importance of your weight loss goals. It is akin to holding yourself back from success.

Understand when and when not to make compromises. But also, know that your IF lifestyle should not affect other aspects of your life adversely. Your social life shouldn't suffer because you are trying to lose extra weight. Your loved ones should also understand your journey and endeavor to make compromises of their own when necessary.

The second rule is "undertake." This essentially means taking over the execution of any planned, upcoming social events with family or friends. Doing this gives you more control over what you consume at such events. Also, you can use that opportunity to choose activities that cannot affect your fasting window.

Fortunately, intermittent fasting itself is a flexible diet, which means that you just need to tweak a little here and there whenever necessary. If you follow the 16:8 plan, that makes life even easier for you.

Finally, "explain" means you should outrightly tell friends and family whenever you are on a fast. Sometimes, explaining what you are doing is the key to getting them to accommodate your new lifestyle. You can even introduce interested loved ones to fasting. Having a group of people interested in the same thing can make a difference in your life as you become increasingly acclimatized to extended fasting.

Once you get them to understand why you are on that journey, they will do their best to support your progress. Don't be surprised when they start sending texts to let you know that your fasting window is still on and you "shouldn't eat that apple!"

And you can find people to fast with. Regardless of the approach you take to fasting, you can quickly get one or two people to fast together.

Conclusion

As you have learned throughout this book, weight loss via intermittent fasting is authentic and achievable. Being a woman in your 50s, losing weight need not be an arduous task. You can reap tons of benefits from fasting, and weight loss is just one of those benefits. Finding an approach suitable for you is as simple as ABC, thanks to the many intermittent fasting variations.

All you need to succeed in your intermittent fasting journey is to stick to everything you have learned in this book. Follow every rule, tip, and technique diligently, and you might just become the fittest 50-year-old lady you have ever come across. Good luck!

Here's another book by Daron McClain that you might like

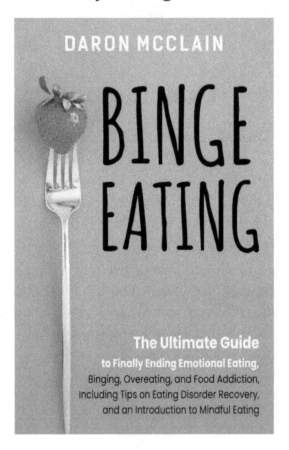

DARON MCCLAIN

BINGE EATING

The Ultimate Guide
to Finally Ending Emotional Eating,
Binging, Overeating, and Food Addiction,
Including Tips on Eating Disorder Recovery,
and an Introduction to Mindful Eating

References

CenterForDiscoveryED. (2019, February 5). The Dangers of Intermittent Fasting - Center For Discovery. Center for Discovery. https://centerfordiscovery.com/blog/the-dangers-of-intermittent-fasting

Chuang, J.-C., & Zigman, J. M. (2010). Ghrelin's Roles in Stress, Mood, and Anxiety Regulation. *International Journal of Peptides*, *2010*. https://www.hindawi.com/journals/ijpep/2010/460549/

Collier, R. (2013). Intermittent fasting: the science of going without. Canadian Medical Association Journal, 185(9), E363–E364. https://www.cmaj.ca/content/185/9/E363

Crane, M. M., Jeffery, R. W., & Sherwood, N. E. (2016). Exploring Gender Differences in a Randomized Trial of Weight Loss Maintenance. American Journal of Men's Health, 11(2), 369–375.

de Cabo, R., & Mattson, M. P. (2019). Effects of Intermittent Fasting on Health, Aging, and Disease. *New England Journal of Medicine*, *381*(26), 2541–2551. https://www.nejm.org/doi/10.1056/NEJMra1905136

Research on intermittent fasting shows health benefits. (2020, February 27). National Institute on Aging. https://www.nia.nih.gov/news/research-intermittent-fasting-shows-health-benefits

Stockman, M.-C., Thomas, D., Burke, J., & Apovian, C. M. (2018). Intermittent Fasting: Is the Wait Worth the Weight? Current Obesity Reports, 7(2), 172–185. https://link.springer.com/article/10.1007/s13679-018-0308-9

Tello, M. (2018, June 26). Intermittent fasting: Surprising update - Harvard Health Blog. Harvard Health Blog. https://www.health.harvard.edu/blog/intermittent-fasting-surprising-update-2018062914156

CPSIA information can be obtained
at www.ICGtesting.com
Printed in the USA
BVHW012144140322
631502BV00002B/86